# Are You Sure
## What You're Eating?

# The Poisoning
# of
# America

## What Every Digestive Sufferer

## Should Know

### By: Nancie Paruso

# Dedication

### Dr. Leon Neiman

I am dedicating this book to Dr. Leon Neiman of Akron, Ohio. Dr. Neiman is a well-respected ENT specialist and a doctor far ahead of his time.

Over 25 years ago, he taught me to understand the wonders of the human body and its ability to heal itself. His belief was that food not only nourished us, but could also heal us. He was and is a Doctor who uses diet, proper hydration, and vitamins to assist in healing his patients. He uses pharmaceuticals only when it is necessary on a patient-to-patient basis. I had forgotten his words and wisdom from over 25 years ago but I have found my direction again and I have incorporated that knowledge he shared with me in this book.

God bless you!

In addition, I would like to thank my "Family" physician, Doctor Leonard Wojnowich for believing in me and for taking my ragged book outline and reading it. Letting me know I had something of value to share. He is a great "Doctor" in Savannah and I high recommend him to anyone.

A special thank you to Karen McBride and Dr. L Curtsinger for encouraging me to put my journey down on paper so I could share it with others—it provided me with hope of helping someone else who is experiencing the same issues.

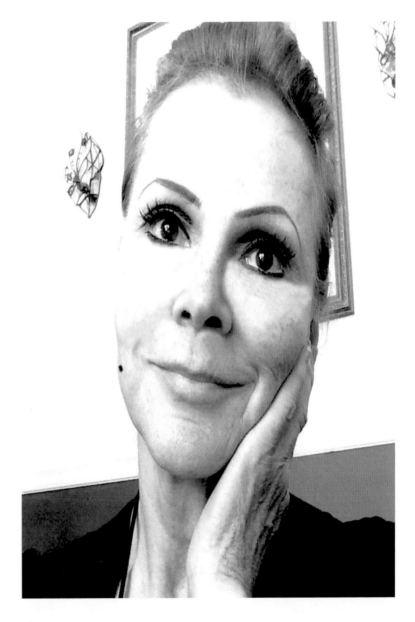

NO DIET BOOK, DIET PILL, DIET PLAN, CLEANSE, OR CLEANSE PRODUCT WILL EVER BE THE ANSWER. FOR A HEALTHY DIGESTIVE SYSTEM— THESE ARE TEMPORARY MEASURES.

YOU MUST CHANGE WHAT YOU EAT—THAT IS THE BOTTOM LINE AND THAT IS WHAT I FOUND OUT ON MY JORNEY AND MY SUBSQUENT WAY BACK TO HEALTH—AND A LIFE WITH QUALITY!

WE ARE CURRENTLY OVER-MEDICATED; YOUR ANSWER TO FEELING BETTER IS NOT ONE PILL AFTER ANOTHER. MEDICATION GENERALLY WILL NOT BE THE ANSWER TO YOUR DIGESTIVE AND IMMUNE ISSUES—IT TREATS THE SYMPTOMS NOT YOUR ROOT CAUSE. IT IS SIMPLE—YOU NEED TO MAKE A DECISION AND BE RESPONSIBLE FOR A GREAT DEAL OF YOUR HEALTH.—THAT MEANS YOU NEED TO STOP EATING PROCESSED FOODS—PERIOD!.

EDUCATE YOURSELF AND YOU AND YOUR "FAMILY" WILL BE HEALTHY TOGETHER

THERE IS NO LIFE IF YOU DON'T HAVE THE QUALITY OF LIFE THAT ALLOWS YOU TO LIVE! THERE ARE "NO" DO-OVERS. GET IT RIGHT AND GET IT RIGHT NOW FOR THE SAKE OF YOUR FAMILY AND YOUR OWN HEALTH!

This is my personal "Journal" it is my journey into digestive hell, my experiences, my research, my diagnosis and finally my path on how I found a way to reclaim my life.

It is a collection of daily journal entries, research and research articles that provided me with a path back to digestive health.

My researched was recorded to help me find out what was wrong with me. I suffered for 2 ½ years with a digestive problem of unknown origin. I was responsible for finding my own diagnosis and for researching what I needed to do to find my way back to health. Very honestly, this started out as a path for "just" my needs. During the research process, I found out that thousands of people both children and adults were fighting with health issues that presented the same or similar symptoms.

Although this is my medical journal, I found it challenging to provide a title that would reach all those who could benefit from this information that I collected during my research and diagnosis process. Where I was covering mainly digestive issues I found many health issues were overlapping and one name didn't convey my findings. However, the multiple health issues I have included are connected by one single commonality—what we eat.

Friends and family encouraged me to share my story and my research so others would have a chance to find their diagnosis.

My story covers my journey, which was and is primarily a digestive issue, but also includes so much more information and affects so many other escalating health issues.

I have touched on the following issues, Depression, Obesity, Type II Diabetes, Autism, Brain-Gut connection, Alzheimer's, and our overall poor health as a nation.

My research is solid and the confusion I chronicle is unfortunately too true in regards to the issue of High Fructose Corn Syrup, GMO's and Trans Fats. I was a naysayer in the past—but I am healthy today only due to the fact I made a conscious decision to change

I condensed my daily journal version because my research had reached 3,000+ pages as I searched to find my own Diagnosis. As mentioned before it includes my personal medical records.

I will explain how I found out what was wrong with me, what research took place and why this (Digestive issues) seems to be such a difficult process when it comes to a diagnosis.

This is not a miracle; I have no medication to push, no magic pill, cleansing product or gimmick. Simply put it is how I found my way back to good health. I am sharing this with you to encourage education and share a process that will help you and bring increased awareness to our health crisis in America.

People will never truly understand something until it happens to them!

Just remember, "Educating yourself does not mean that you were stupid in the first place; it means that you are intelligent enough to know that there is plenty left to learn." Not my quote it is from "I flipping love science."

My purpose for publishing my Health Journal, a blog an email or a text in regards to Fructose/HFCS is to heighten awareness to the dangers of processed food.

In case you haven't noticed conversations about bowel movements and vomiting aren't the page-turners they use to be! I remain driven to increase awareness and the removal of food additives. Education is the main reason I decided to share all that I had learned.

I have no product to sell but I have accurate and precise education I want to disseminate it to as many as possible to try to cut off the avalanche of poor health in this country.

If you read, comprehend, and decide you are going to eat whatever you want anyway—that is your choice but you need to know the facts before you continue to poison your system or that of your families!

The Poisoning of America isn't just about what is in our food. It is how the advertising, pharmaceutical, food conglomerates and medical industry continue to create confusion instead of providing honest answers.

## Do you want to improve the quality of your life?

This information in this book can provide you with the means needed to achieve a positive and healthier you!

No one can understand your pain and frustration better than someone who has walked in your shoes.

I spent my days in pain, depression, frustration, bloating, and nausea I no longer had control of anything in my life!

I researched out of necessity due to the fact I was desperate to find a Diagnosis to my own health issue.

What I found provided me with a diagnosis. However, it wasn't just a diagnosis for me; it was a diagnosis for *thousands*.

What would it mean to you if you were no longer hampered by your health issues? How would you like to look and feel younger? How much better off would you be if you had mental clarity, increased energy, and less anxiety? Those changes are possible now.

*This is your turning point. All the symptoms you are experiencing may seem separate but there is a link!*

Our bodies are in a constant state of chronic inflammation and modern medicine knows that inflammation is the underlying cause for so many of health issues we face today. We all have a boiling point…I have reached mine…when will you reach yours?

Our brains and bodies have been and continue to be hijacked, since the 60's, by processed foods and Genetically Modified Organisms. (GMO) which we eat every time you eat processed foods. Please note once again that this is a condensed version of my daily journal and research that I used in providing myself with a diagnosis and maybe paraphrased in order to provide an affordable resource but keeping the correct medical facts!

I was the test subject and I tested each food on my charts….and often suffered the consequences if I selected something that was hard to digest.

## Expectations: What it can mean to you!

Note: These were my personal results and everyone's results will vary according to how you modify your life-style and how many food intolerances you have. This is what I did.

- I quit every beverage or food product that was even connected to High Fructose Corn Syrup or natural *fructose* cold turkey
- Within the first week, I started to feel better and the pain started to get bearable
- By the end of week two, I noticed the bloating, gas and nausea was dissipating
- Week three my depression started to diminish…at least enough that, I could tell the difference.
- After 30 days of eating from my food list, I had lost 25 pounds.

- PLEASE NOTE: THE WEIGHT LOSS HAD NOTHING TO DO WITH IMAGE...IT HAD EVERYTHING TO DO WITH HEALTH. I HAD GAINED 50 POUNDS IN NINE WEEKS AT THE BEGINNING OF THIS HEALTH ISSUE.
- I stopped taking several of the medications, and never reached the level of intestinal debilitation again
- After 65 days on myself created Fructose-Specific Food program, I had lost over 50 pounds. My memory was much improved and nothing seemed as fuzzy as it once had
- Six months after the initial start of eating my selected foods, I found that my life was completely changed. I no longer was fatigued, angry, or achy

None of the changes ever took place while I was on medication or under the care of my specialist. Every health improvement I experienced—was and is strictly based on an urgent need to change my diet.

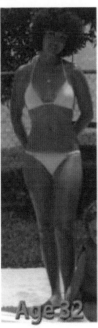 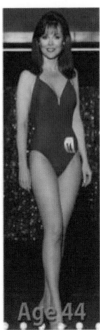 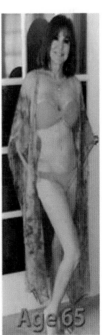

Many people believe that to empower one with the understanding of their own health is a life- altering event, it was for me, and I wanted to share that feeling with everyone!

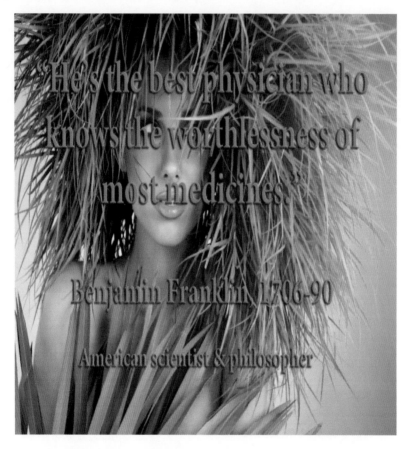

"He's the best physician who knows the worthlessness of most medicines."

Benjamin Franklin 1706-90

American scientist & philosopher

Note to all ER Physicians and GI Specialists

First, Do No Harm!

## A word to all doctor's—whether it is an ER, Hospitalist, or GI Specialist—listen to your patients.

I recently had a chance to see a friend/doctor and I told him of a recent hospital incident regarding a TIA I had experienced and that the drugs for the episode was going to create problems for my digestive tract. Obviously, I would have taken what would have saved my life if my life had been in the balance but I am very protective of my Digestive System.

He then told me to make sure I never ask for a specific pain med...because whether it is fair or not the ER thinks drug seeker immediately and will and does treat you with that "thought process", the need to read up on the recent work done by the University of Oklahoma and other studies.

He (my doctor) said it is sad that for those who need help and that help being very specific to the patient's body chemistry—live in fear of sharing that information because they will be labeled as a drug seeker...not a person in pain who is dealing with a very real health issue.

I have not researched my brain issue regarding my TIA. However, my gut—well—no one knows it better than me—I have been able to diagnosis, replicate the problems, heal myself by eating properly, and repeat this for the sake of peer review discussion. There is no cure but you can take control.

I know that there is a connection between the Brain and Gut—I am not moving into neurosurgery...I bow to their knowledge and experience but you need to make sure that your doctor knows you have more than one issue going on in your body.

Remember what might help one issue could be a disaster for the other issue. It has now been 4 days since I have been home. Today was the first day that my gut seemed to be close to going back to "normal!"

Experiencing a TIA had a strong impact on me—but due to the fact I was not being heard I suffered a 4 day episode with my Fructose Malabsorption issue—along with the worry about experiencing another TIA episode.

DOCTORS LISTEN TO YOUR PATIENTS! WE AR NOT LOOKING FOR PAIN MEDIATION WE ARE SIMPLY TRYING TO HEAD-OFF AN ANOTHER DIRE HEALTH ISSUE.

To all Doctor's you can't assume patients are seeking pain medications that by telling you what other issues you have and how you react to medication is important for all of you doctors to hear. It doesn't matter if you are an ER Doctor or a Hospitalist assigned to a patient you need to stop branding and penalizing the patient for telling you what has worked without side effects and what creates more health issues for the patient. Re-evaluate your approach!

If a patient was providing the ER with medications, they are allergic to—the medical staff doesn't blink an eye—if the patient tells them that due to other health issues certain drugs including pain medications affect them in a very negative way—well then you are screwed! Regardless of your medical history and experience, you don't dare mention pain medication—why is this so taboo?

If the patients know, certain drugs provide negative issues for their digestive illness why should you penalize them for sharing relevant information.

All of those who are patients know what reaction you will experience so why are we punished for relating honest information.

People in Pain need help. It is not our fault that people in the medical profession see the other side of the coin—that being drug seekers and/or attention seekers—but doctors should not punish you for being honest and sharing pertinent information that can impact the health of the patient!

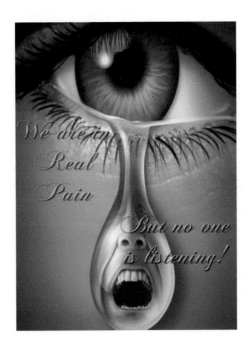

Learn to listen to what is being said!

**Irritable Bowel Syndrome (IBS), Extreme Fatigue,
Autism, Alzheimer's Disease
GERD/Acid Reflux, FODMAPS, Gastritis Support,
Obesity, Type II Diabetes, Hereditary Fructose
Intolerance, Candida, Leaky Gut, Depression, Gluten
Chronic Inflammation, Lactose, Celiac, and
Autoimmune Health Issues**

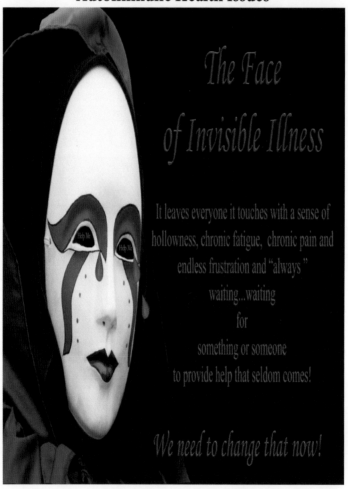

These so called "Invisible Diseases" are not Invisible to thousands!

All medical professionals please treat us as individuals and don't lump us up into one big ball.

Any Doctor who assumes that a patient in pain is just a drug seeker—well, they need re-evaluate their thought process and realize 90% of all people they see are not looking for a "fix."

We are individuals with our own unique body chemistry—we are not just a group of people to be lumped together we should be treated independently with respect and dignity because we deserve nothing less.

So, shame on the Medical Professionals that don't look at us as unique individuals who need their help—instead you—the ER or Hospitalist jump to conclusions that increase the frustration and pain of patients who are in very REAL pain. You are our judge jury and hangman—it is too easy for you the medical professionals—simply to label a person as a drug seeker than it is to find the root or our illnesses.

Because of this attitude, there are thousands of honest individuals who are not looking for attention and not seeking drugs—and are not being treated as they should be treated because of this mind set.

Each patient is an individual and should not be lumped into a group for the sake of a quick and easy way for Emergency Room Doctor's to get through their workload.

Be Smart!  Live Healthy!

## Disclosure

This book is comprised of my health journal, personal medical records, and 3,000+ pages of research that I have compiled on each of my 12 diagnoses. All information is from valid Medical Universities/Research Centers, medical books and articles. Any article that needed a citation is properly marked. The result of my research was finding my own diagnosis. The information collected through her person research correlates with several top Gastroenterologists. The food charts (Copyright Pending) meet and exceed the standard.

It took several months of research to provide the information that I have condensed. It is solid medical research and not medical industry research—which is a big difference.

It is possible for any individual to take the 2 years+ to accomplish the same thing that I am providing. It is also possible that if you are ill and undiagnosed then you need of direction to good health now and not three+ months from now. I'm providing you with Medical Information and my personal outcome. I'm also sharing over 12 digestive issues with you and direction to where you may find your exact match. It is important to me that regain your health— although we all know there isn't a cure yet.

The basis of her book is from her personal experience, frustration, and finally her diagnosis through education.

Graphics: All graphics created by: Nancie Paruso

Graphics: Copyright 2013 pending

Background pictures are of my own medical scans, personal pictures and purchased background pictures providing me with legal rights to use them in my book, website or Blog.

Cover design Copyright pending 2013 by Nancie Paruso

You will be amazed at how good you can feel!

Don't Suffer in Silence one more day!

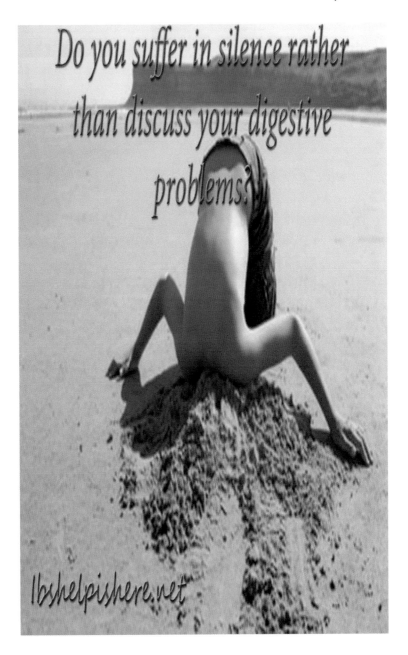

"This book has information that I think every patient out there who has been diagnosed with the nonspecific "Irritable Bowel Syndrome" label needs to know.  I am a physician who has been in practice for more than 20 years, and I consider myself one who thinks "out of the box", yet there were many things I learned from Nancie and her incredible fight to find answers and regain her health. This book and her information need to be in the hands of every gastroenterologist! Bravo Nancie!" - *Dr. Carmelita Fields of Savannah, Georgia*

"Nancie's desperate search for answers clearly indicates the necessity of the medical community to explore outside of the "box" for solutions to perplexing symptomatology. This book is a must-read for anyone struggling with a mystery illness." - *Peggy Wendt, Holistic Health, and Wellness (review on Amazon)*

"I can attest to most of the facts in this book. My wife has suffered with bloating, diarrhea, and PAIN for over thirty years. Therefore, I think I am somewhat of an expert. My Wife has been to many doctors and tried all of the different cures also avoiding salads in restaurants and whatever advice they had. Finally, a friend introduced my wife to Nancie Paruso. She told Ruth my wife that she had been suffering with the same symptoms too.  After some advice from Nancie, the bloating stopped the next day. Some adjustment in her diet and checking all the food she used for FRUCTOSE ended years of suffering for her and me.  We just received a signed copy of the book as Nancie was writing it when we got her advice .My wife went to the doctors today and told her about her cure. The doc did not believe her. I can tell you it WORKS. Get the book and read it." - *Frank Van Giesen (review on Amazon)*

"Technically, my diagnosis was IBS. Come to find out I had SIBO, Fructose Malabsorption and food sensitivities. You can change your life!

If your or anyone else in your family has suffered for years, months, or even days then it has been too long. I myself followed Nancie's advice and plan on taking it steps further. I am going to fight like hell to make sure my husband and four children don't become another statistic. I beg you! Share this book with everyone you know! This is not the end but the beginning!" - *Jessica Nelson, wife and mother (review on Amazon)*

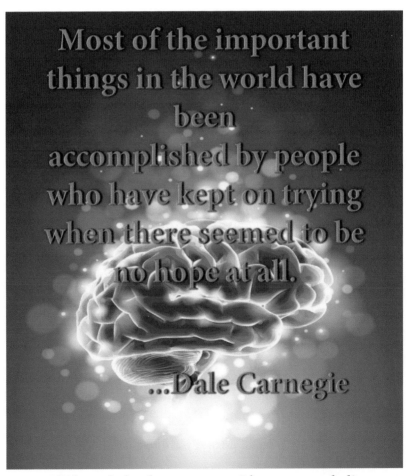

Most of the important things in the world have been accomplished by people who have kept on trying when there seemed to be no hope at all.

...Dale Carnegie

If I have helped one person, I have succeeded!

# Introduction

By sharing this information with you my hope is to help you avoid an avalanche of many illnesses that currently affect both you and your children. We are currently on a path of poor health of epidemic proportions.

I have written this book (actually it is the complete journal I kept of my illness and my life for over 3 years) after a prolonged struggle to discover an accurate diagnosis for my digestive health problem, and its effective treatment. My credentials for writing this book would be my 4 years of dealing with this *"Health Issue"* and months of research to find my own diagnosis.

My biggest challenge in writing this book was taking my daily journal and trying to create a format that would compel you to want to read all of my facts and findings. My research is sound and my story is true and "one" word did change my life.

Two and a half years after the onset of my illness, I was on my way to becoming a professional patient. All the drugs, ER visits, doctor's appointments, and hospital admissions were simply treating my symptoms, not my illness. Had I continued down that path, I would not have survived to write my story for you.

The research I am sharing with you is information that can be substantiated by several major hospital/university centers, finally narrowing it down to four. It is acknowledged and validated by several top Gastroenterologists who are well respected throughout their community, as well as, our country.

I have touched on a dozen digestive health issues and a half dozen of other issues that are associated with my illness.

However, there are so many other digestive issues I didn't touch on in this book—such as Gerd (Acid Reflux), Dumping Syndrome, lactose intolerance, Candida Diet individuals, Celiac/Coeliac disease, and multiple food allergies. I encourage all of you to educate yourself so you and your family can live healthy lives!

In the end, I was responsible for discovering my own diagnosis!

# Table of Contents

Dedication......................................................................... 2

Forward & About the Author.................................... 3

Note to all ER Physicians and GI Specialists ........... 10

**Disclosure**...................................................... **16**

Testimonials.................................................. 18

Introduction................................................. 20

Chapter One: How it All Began............................. 29

Chapter Two: My Descent into Confusion ................. 31

Chapter Three:  Eleven Different Diagnoses ............. 35

**My First Diagnosis:  Colonic Ileus**........................**35**

**My Second Diagnosis:  Bowel Blockage**................**35**

**Fibromyalgia**..................................................**38**

**Adhesions**......................................................**39**

**Narcotic Ileus**................................................**39**

**SIBO** ..............................................................**43**

**Leaky Gut Syndrome** ......................................**44**

**Telescoping Intestine** .....................................**44**

**Ulcerative Colitis and Crohn's Disease** ...............**45**

**My Eleventh Diagnosis: Irritable Bowel Syndrome** .................**49**

**VAGUS NERVE AND MESENTERIC VEIN** ...............**51**

Vasovagal Reflex ........................................ 51

What are intestinal ischemic syndromes?.................55

What causes these syndromes? ...........................55

Are these conditions more common at a certain age?.............55

Types of Intestinal Ischemic Syndromes .......................... 55

Chapter Four: The "Negative" Impact of Unrelenting Pain ..... 57

**Early Pain Theories and Remedies** ........................................... 57

**Unrelieved Pain Has Consequences—There Are Many Adverse Effects of Unrequited Acute Pain** ............................................ 57

History of "Oligoanalgesia" ........................................................ 59

**The Importance of Pain Control** ............................................. 60

**Uncontrolled pain can:** ............................................................. 61

**Understanding Pain—Gate Theory of Pain** ............................ 61

**The Peripheral Nervous System** ............................................. 62

**Breaking the Pain-Tension Cycle** ............................................ 63

**Stress Pain Cycle** ..................................................................... 63

**Debunking Pain Myths** ............................................................ 65

Establishing Trust with Your Health Care Team ...................... 66

**The Costs of Pain** ..................................................................... 66

**The Personal Burdens of Pain** ................................................ 67

**The Impact of Pain on Friends and Family** ............................ 67

**The Financial Costs of Pain** .................................................... 68

**Abstract** ................................................................................... 68

**Emergency Room and your Gut** ............................................. 69

Principles of Pain Assessment and Causes of Under-Treatment of Acute Pain ............................................................................ 69

**Chronic Pain Fact Sheet/by Marcia E. Bedard, PhD** ............. 71

**Pain Often Undertreated** ........................................................ 73

Chapter Five: The Word That Changed My Life ...................... 77

**Finally a Diagnosis and Direction** ........................................... 80

**What is Hereditary Fructose Intolerance?** ............................. 81

Hereditary fructose intolerance (HFI) symptoms:.................. 82

Sensitivity.................................................................................. 82

Testing...this information, I read in the paper that Dr. Satish Rao Published. He is located in Augusta Georgia and if you have insurance or the cash, Dr. Rao is the person who will help you! .................................................................................................... 83

Treatment ............................................................................... 85

Cure .......................................................................................... 85

Chapter Six: Identify, Educate & Eradicate ........................... 92

Definition of Fructose Malabsorption: ............................... 98

Isn't Fructose Natural? ........................................................... 98

What is High Fructose Corn Syrup? ..................................... 99

How is HFCS Produced?.......................................................... 99

Why & When Was High Fructose Corn Syrup (HFCS) Introduced to Our Food? ..................................................... 100

Does HFCS Come in Different Strengths? ......................... 101

What Synonyms Does The Sugar Industry Use For HFCS When Labeling? ................................................................... 102

I Have IBS...How Does That Relate to Fructose Malabsorption? .................................................................... 103

Symptoms of Fructose Malabsorption that Mirror HFI: ........ 104

How do "Our" Bodies Absorb Fructose?.......................... 105

Chapter Seven: HFCS & Your Body!.....................................106

How Does Fructose Malabsorption /HFCS Affect The Body?.. 107

Is HFCS Harmful to Our Body? ........................................... 107

Which Organs Are Affected First When Ingesting HFCS?........ 107

HFCS Creates Chronic Inflammation which is a Corner Stone for Cancer ................................................................................... 109

Type II Diabetes ..................................................................... 121

Insulin Resistance ........................................... 122

What is Glycation? ........................................... 122

How does AGE's affect our Aging? ........................ 123

Aging ........................................................... 123

Liver ............................................................ 125

Kidney/Fructose ............................................. 126

Obesity/Fructose ............................................ 127

Depression/Fructose ........................................ 128

Uric Acid Levels as a Marker for Fructose Toxicity ..... 132

What Are AGEs? Advanced Glycation End ................ 132

What Do AGEs Do In The Body? ........................... 133

How Do I Protect Myself? .................................. 133

Chapter Eight: HFCS Number One Enemy! ................ 137

What reason does the Corn Industry have of misleading the public? ...................................................... 139

What Does Science Have to Say About HFCS? ........... 140

Five Reasons HFCS Can Kill You! ......................... 141

Accountability Status –- Currently None! ................ 147

Chapter Nine: The Missing Link to Good Health .......... 150

The Brain-Gut Connection in IBS and Fructose Malabsorption. ................................................ 151

How our Gut Influences our Mood...Mental Health ..... 155

Autism and Fructose ........................................ 155

Alzheimer's Disease and Fructose ........................ 158

Research is On Going or is it? ............................. 161

Fructose is the Next "Gluten Epidemic" on the Horizon! ....... 161

Chapter Ten: Additional Concerns! ........................ 165

Fiber ................................................................................. 166

Caloric Content .................................................................. 166

Use in Foods ...................................................................... 166

Inulin in Processed Foods .................................................. 166

Remember Inulin is Another Word for Fructose! ................. 167

Probiotics and Prebiotics ................................................... 170

Sorbitol---Yet, another Concern! ........................................ 171

Chapter Eleven: Eliminate IBS & Fructose ............................ 174

A Calorie Has Never Been Just a Calorie ............................ 175

How High Fructose Corn Syrup has and is Decimating Human
Health. ............................................................................... 176

Carbs: Never Too Low! ....................................................... 177

How Much Fructose Are You Consuming? ........................... 178

Fructose-Specific Food Charts ............................................ 179

Acidity Factor in Your Diet! ................................................ 182

Chapter Twelve:  Fructose-Specific Food Charts .................... 183

Fructose-Specific Food Charts ............................................ 184

Sweeteners ......................................................................... 197

Alcohol: .............................................................................. 207

A protein and fat breakfast, e.g. bacon and eggs, does not produce rapid hunger, because it does not produce a large insulin rise and glucose fall.
Chapter Thirteen:   You Are Never "Cured" .......................................................................... 210

Chapter Fourteen:   Sugar GMO's & Labeling ....................... 216

Autoimmune and More ....................................................... 221

Odds & Ends, GMO's & Labeling ........................................ 226

What is a GMO and How Does  it Affect Us? ....................... 226

Uses ................................................................................... 227

GM Crops ...................................................... 228

6 Negative Side Affects to Eating Genetically Modified Foods 230

Are you Consuming the nine Most Genetically Modified Foods?
................................................................... 232

Chapter Fifteen: The Poisoning of America............................236

Advertising, Food Conglomerates, Pharmaceuticals, Medical
Profession .......................................................... 236

A Flaw in Our Thought Process? ........................................ 240

Chapter Sixteen: The Debate Rages On...................................243

Nancie Paruso Hyper-sensitive Theory ................................. 243

Environmental Destruction ............................................. 248

Health Consequences.................................................... 249

Food Supply at Risk.................................................... 250

Read, Comprehend, You Decide! ......................................... 251

Sloan Kettering:....................................................... 251

High Fructose Corn Syrup and interesting ways to create
pandemics. Part 1...................................................... 251

Pancreatic cancers use high fructose corn syrup (HFCS),
common in the Western diet to fuel their growth ................... 252

High Fructose Corn Syrup Direct Correlation with Autism in
the U.S. – Clinic Epigenetics. 2012 .............................. 255

Sweeteners Tags: American Psychiatric Association, ASD,
Autism spectrum, Epidemiology of autism, Health, High-
fructose corn syrup, Northeastern University, United States. 255

Heat forms potentially harmful substance in high-fructose corn
syrup: Hydroxymethylfurfural (HMF) (39) ........................... 255

University Of Southern California and Oxford Researchers Find
High Fructose Corn Syrup-Global Prevalence of Diabetes Link!
................................................................... 257

**Cannabis Less Addicting Than High Fructose Corn Syrup!** ...... **261**

The Top 13 Most Addictive Substances .................................... 262

**Is Sugar Toxic?** ..................................................... **268**

**New York Times Article on Robert Lustig Sugar** .................... **268**

**My Challenge to You– Patient, Parent, or Spouse!** ............... **278**

Chapter Seventeen: GI Specialists & Our Digestive Decline....280

**This is my challenge to each doctor!** ........................... **282**

**Sugar/Fructose & Medicine** ..................................... **283**

Chapter Eighteen: Reclaim your Health ............................284

**Resources to Change Your Life!** ............................... **284**

**Your Expectations & Results** .................................... **290**

Chapter Nineteen: What Your Eyes Say About Your Health..292

**And the possible link between your Gut and Cholesterol Plaque.**
.................................................................. **292**

**HOW FOOD ADDITIVES TIE INTO THE INCREASE OF
HOLLENHORST PLAQUE** .......................................... **294**

**How can your Gut Affect our Eyes?** ............................ **296**

Special and Sincere Thanks! .....................................306

Disclaimer: .....................................................307

Works Cited .....................................................309

Appendices .....................................................317

SIBO - In-depth .................................................317

Leaky Gut-- In-depth ............................................320

Irritable Bowel Syndrome --In depth .............................321

Hereditary Fructose Intolerance -- In-depth .....................322

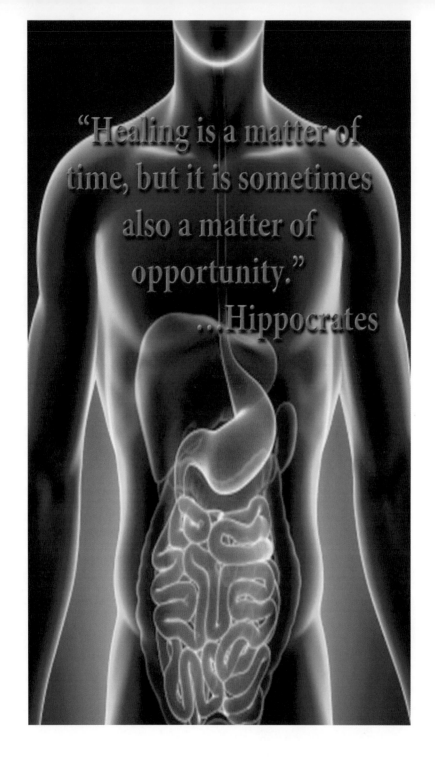

"Healing is a matter of time, but it is sometimes also a matter of opportunity."

...Hippocrates

My nightmare started very suddenly, or so I thought. In retrospect, it was probably coming on slowly over a period of 2 to 3 years. In any case, my illness went full blown around the time of my 60th birthday in October of 2010, when I was rushed to the emergency room. Over the next two and a half years, and 48 visits to the emergency room, my illness escalated into a constant battle with severe bouts of pain, nausea, bloating, rapid weight gain, depression, and the early signs of dementia. Physicians administered over 35 different medications to me, many together with unknown chemical interactions.

During this time, physicians incorrectly diagnosed me with eleven different intestinal health illnesses. I now found myself back right where I started, I was still extremely ill. Emergency room doctors and staff had begun to perceive me as simply an individual who wanted either attention or drugs! Moreover, they treated me that way. The upshot is that I diligently researched and became intimately acquainted with each of these eleven diagnoses. I learned as much as I could about every one of them, with a firm belief that each was the correct diagnosis. I then set out, on my own, to find my true diagnosis.

I want to share with you what I learned on my journey to reclaim my health, and to assist you in alleviating your suffering from the catchall diagnosis *irritable bowel syndrome*. I will walk you through each diagnosis I was given, one by one, since many of these issues have overlapping symptoms, and are difficult to differentiate. Some of you may be embarrassed to talk about your symptoms with doctors. I have found no doctor/hospital sanctioned support groups for people who suffer from the symptoms discussed in this book.

You need not suffer in silence, because you are not alone!

By the end of this book, I will have explained to you where I started, where my research led me, and how I found answers, which finally brought me back to health.

I would like to state for the record that I am not a doctor, nurse, or dietician, nor do I work in the medical field. I am a 63-year-old female patient, and I share my story here, based on my medical files and literally thousands of pages of research. I would like to make it clear that I have immense respect for the majority of the medical profession. I do not mean to slander or malign the profession in any way. However, keep in mind that even health professionals can make mistakes.

The digestive health issue from which I was suffering is a health issue that affects thousands of people.

Our medical professionals, however, lack awareness and knowledge about it. I discovered, in fact, that certain manufactured ingredients common to the average American diet were the cause of my suffering. These ingredients put my life in a virtual tailspin for two and a half years. Yet, they are contained in foods and beverages today in increasing quantity. You should be aware of these ingredients, and learn whether they may be causing your irritable bowel syndrome. I was astounded, and empowered, by this discovery, and believe you may be too!

"Now, good digestion waits on appetite and health on both!"

...William Shakespeare

That first trip to the emergency room in October of 2010 marked the beginning of my descent into confusion. What I thought would be a short-term event marked the beginning of a long, confusing, and humiliating descent into a valley from which I did not emerge for two and a half years.

The first night I was rushed to the hospital, I was in agony with tremendous stomach pain, I was nauseated, and my stomach was extremely bloated. The teams of doctors at the onset my health crisis were specialists, who ran numerous tests to determine the cause of my problem. Each doctor would examine me, and try to provide an explanation for my problem. Unfortunately, they were unsure what the cause was. Doctors alleviated my pain by administering large amounts of pain medication, and were concerned about the condition of my colon. Doctors said the extreme bloating (I looked nine months pregnant!) was due to a large number of air loops in my intestines, which could endanger my life.

This is an x-ray image which shows how painfully distended my stomach had become.

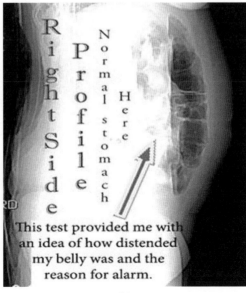

This test provided me with an idea of how distended my belly was and the reason for alarm.

31

My first concern was the pain and relentless nausea.

I found myself in a fog, whether it was from my illness, or the medication was not clear to me at the time. After my symptoms subsided, they sent me home, still in a mental fog, and loaded with an arsenal of 18 different medications.

I soon found that I would add another concern to my growing list of symptoms: rapid weight gain. Within the next 8 to 9 weeks, I gained 50 pounds! I had never weighed more than 110 pounds, and always wore a petite size. However, my weight gain was not simply a concern because of vanity. My weight gain was sudden and not gradual…there was not time to adjust I became acutely aware of new limitations when walking, sitting, or bending over. I was out of breath, and tired easily. I was beginning to balloon.

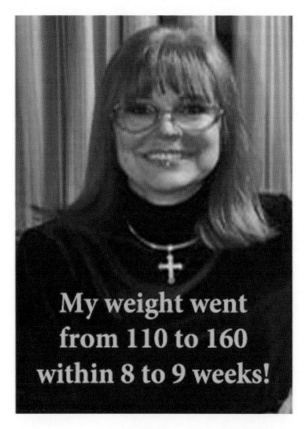

I was now weighing in at an impossible 160 pounds. Sometimes, I would gain still more weight daily from bloating.

Bloat might add 10 to 12 more pounds a day, making life more miserable. Doctors could not explain why this was happening.

My new weight caused a profound lack of energy, and left me lethargic. I became depressed, and before long, I resigned myself to staying at home. I only left the house to go to the doctor or the hospital. I would look at myself in the mirror and could not recognize the person looking back. I was bloated beyond words, my color was ashen, and side effects from the medication were only compounding the issue.

As if that was not enough, another humiliating adjustment, and the main reason for not leaving the house now, was my need to stay close to the bathroom. I was beginning to have extremely embarrassing "emergencies." Incontinence was a stunning adjustment for me, because I had always been fit and had led an active life! I no longer had control of all of my bodily functions. It was necessary to stay home, until I could adjust. I now found myself in unfamiliar territory and in sudden need Depends.

With no insurance and doctors' bills mounting up, my stress increased. The pressure of not knowing what was wrong with me only added to that stress, and to that of my poor husband. Every time I had an episode that sent me to the hospital, a little voice kept telling me I was creating more financial problems. With work out of the question due to incontinence and pain, our financial future was in jeopardy.

Lastly, depression was beginning to take hold of me, and I was reluctant to get off the couch. I would lie curled up on the couch in our family room where it was dark and quiet. I had reached a point where I was prone to panic attacks if I moved from that safe place.

Ultimately, after 24 months, my symptoms had not changed and this was the list of my symptoms:

- bloating
- diarrhea and/or constipation
- flatulence
- stomach pain, from mild/chronic to acute/erratic
- nausea
- vomiting
- early signs of clinical depression
- aching eyes
- fatigue
- rapid weight gain or loss
- symptoms of hypoglycemia: sugar craving, tremor, fainting

In the next chapter, I will discuss each of the eleven diagnoses I received before discovering my own diagnosis. It may help you to understand each of them, to determine the cause of your own digestive health issue. It may be helpful to you, and to your doctor, if you are familiar with these diagnoses, and their causes. Now, bear with me in this next chapter. It contains a lot of medical information. This knowledge, however, may be helpful to your improved digestive health. I read a quote recently that said, "…to empower one with the understanding of their own health is a life-altering event!" I have indeed found this to be true, in my own life. In fact, you may learn how to alleviate your irritable bowel syndrome by what you read here. You may indeed find it surprising how certain manufactured substances added to our food and beverages are causing an epidemic of digestive health problems in our country.

### My First Diagnosis: Colonic Ileus

After my first admission to the hospital in 2010, doctors diagnosed me with a colonic ileus. I had never heard of this condition. In patient terms, it means paralysis of part of the colon.

In medical terms, an *ileus* is a disruption of the normal propulsive ability of the gastrointestinal tract.

The symptoms of an ileus include, but are not limited to, the following:

- moderate, diffuse abdominal discomfort
- constipation
- abdominal distension
- nausea/vomiting, especially after meals
- vomiting of bile
- lack of bowel movement and/or flatulence
- excessive belching (1)

Your doctor will ask about your symptoms and medical history and perform a physical exam. Diagnosis of an ileus is usually based on symptoms and testing.

### My Second Diagnosis: Bowel Blockage

Later in 2010, when I was rushed to the emergency room again, doctors looked at my chart and saw that I had been admitted the previous month. They drew blood, took me to x-ray, and did a CT scan. The ER provided me with intravenous pain medication, which, by the way, only took the edge off my pain.

The pain was constant, and practically unbearable, unless I was in the hospital with IV medication. Only then did I find respite from the 24/7 pain.

When at home, the medication they had prescribed did little to provide even the slightest relief. It would be months before I found out that I was allergic to it.

Doctors diagnosed me with a bowel blockage, or obstruction. This happens when either your small or large intestine are partially or completely blocked. The blockage prevents food, fluids, and gas from moving through the intestines in the normal way. The blockage may cause severe pain that comes and goes.

Symptoms of a bowel blockage include: (2)

- cramping/stomach pain, often around or below the belly button
- vomiting
- bloating
- constipation/inability to release gas, if the intestine is completely blocked
- diarrhea, if intestine is partially blocked

Each time I went to the ER, I went through the same series of tests. I listed the same symptoms, and all the ER could do was run tests, provide me with some respite from my pain, and send me home with more medications. I had now added the following medications to my home pharmacy: Dicyclomine, Prilosec, Requip, Xanax, and Zyrphen, in addition to the 18 scripts sitting on the counter. I half-heartedly joked that I was on so many pills, that the only thing getting better was the bottom line of the pharmaceutical industry! Unfortunately, in retrospect, there was no "silver bullet" to cure my problem. The pills simply treated the symptoms.

I started asking what the images looked like so I could see the problem. However, the staff at the hospital told me it was difficult for a trained person to understand what they were looking and they felt it would be beyond my comprehension since I was not a medical professional.

My third, fourth, and fifth diagnoses: fibromyalgia, adhesions, and narcotic ileus

In January of 2011, I underwent 7 days of thorough and repeated testing in the hospital. Doctors told me I could possibly have fibromyalgia, with adhesions from past surgeries, and a narcotic ileus brought on by prescription painkillers taken during my hospital admissions.

During this stay, my daughter, who happened to be 7 months pregnant at the time, came to visit. She noticed that my stomach grew substantially larger during the course of the day. In the morning, she would have me stand up, so she could look at my stomach, and compare it to her pregnant belly. By dinnertime, she would again have me stand up next to her, and sure enough, I looked more pregnant than she did. My daughter thought this was noteworthy, and brought it to the attention of a resident, who was on my doctor's staff. The resident agreed that my abdomen had grown significantly, yet he made no note of it on my chart, nor did she mention it to my doctor.

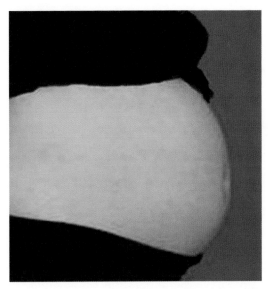

The picture is an actual profile of my stomach in January 2011.

I now had three additional diagnoses added to the first one.

The pain associated with fibromyalgia is often described as a constant dull ache, typically arising from muscles.

Fatigue and sleep disturbances: Patients suffering from fibromyalgia often awaken tired, even though they report sleeping for long periods. Pain frequently disrupts patients' sleep. Many patients with fibromyalgia have other sleep disorders, such as *restless leg syndrome* and *sleep apnea*, which often worsen the symptoms. (3)

Coexisting conditions: Many people who have *fibromyalgia* may also suffer from fatigue, anxiety, depression, endometriosis, headaches, and *irritable bowel syndrome*.

Tests and diagnosis:

In 1990, the American College of Rheumatology (ACR) established two criteria for the diagnosis of fibromyalgia:

- widespread pain lasting at least three months. (Widespread pain affects both sides of the body, above and below the abdomen.)

- at least 11 positive tender points, out of a total possible of 18

However, fibromyalgia symptoms can come and go. In addition, many doctors are uncertain about how much pressure to apply during a tender point exam.

While researchers studying fibromyalgia may still use the 1990 guidelines, doctors in general practice may use less stringent guidelines. These newer diagnostic criteria include:

- Widespread pain lasting at least three months
- No other underlying condition that might be causing the pain

This diagnosis seemed to me like a catchall diagnosis that the medical community provides when they have no other answer! (3)

## Adhesions

Abdominal adhesions cannot be detected by tests or seen through imaging techniques, such as x-rays or ultrasound. Most abdominal adhesions are discovered during surgery. However, abdominal x-rays, a lower gastrointestinal (GI) series, and computerized tomography (CT) scans can diagnose intestinal obstructions. (4)

## Narcotic Ileus

Earlier in this chapter is a description of an ileus, so no need to explain it again here. Your doctor will ask about your symptoms and medical history, and will perform a physical exam.

Doctors based my diagnosis of a possible ileus on their suspicion that I had prior exposure to narcotics. Prior to the onset of this health issue, I was not taking painkillers. I was completely bewildered. The symptoms had not changed. The pain had not changed.

Due to lack of another explanation, it was deemed a problem brought on by pain medication. I felt the doctors were grasping at straws at this point.

All three of these disorders only added to my mounting confusion. These illnesses had vague, diffuse symptoms and required a mountain of medications. I had no concrete information as to why this was happening, and no idea how to alleviate it all! (4)

I was released and sent home with the following medications: Amitriptyline, Zyrtec, Xanax, Amitiza, Atenolol, Prevacid, Albuterol, Flonase, Milk of Magnesia, Colace, Miralax, Levaquin, and Rifaximin. More pills!

Once back home, the same cycle would start all over again: extreme pain, a trip to the ER, then back home, and still no information from the doctors as to why this was happening. I was no further ahead now, than I was after the original onset in October of 2010. Well, as the old adage goes, "The definition of insanity, is doing the same thing repeatedly, expecting different results."

When would this end?

My monthly ER visits continued, but now I was seeing the kind of looks that doctors and staff give to each other when they see you come for the umpteenth time. It was clear that the medical professionals in the ER had begun to consider me a mental patient, or worse.

March came in like a lamb but went out like a lion. I would go through the same tests, they would ask same questions, see the same shadows on the films and scans, and I was sent home more frustrated than before. I no longer believed I would get better, nor could I see light at the end of the tunnel.

Once I called my doctor due to the level of my pain, and his nurse told me they could not treat me at the office, that I needed to go to the ER as I had in the past. She suggested I tell the ER personnel which pain medication worked best on me, so I would be comfortable, as soon as possible. Great, or so I thought!

I found out that by telling the ER that Dilaudid worked best for my pain without negatively affecting my intestinal tract, I was red flagged by the hospital. This meant to staff, it was possible I was just seeking pain meds!

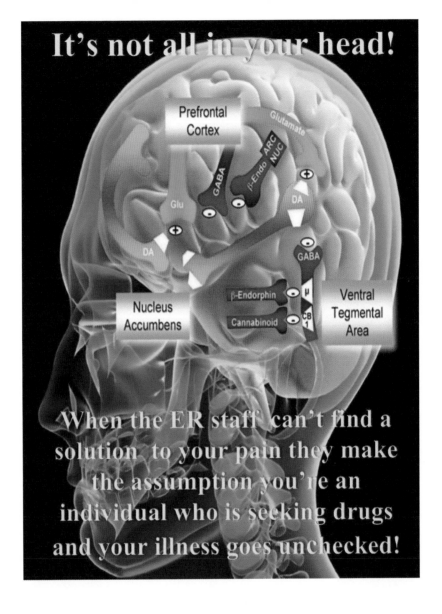

From that point on, I felt that the staff at the emergency room was patronizing me. I believed they no longer looked for the root cause of my health issue. Therefore, I decided to start collecting copies of my medical records, and reading them to see what was going on. Granted, I had to read something 7 times before I could understand anything. Pain meds and other prescriptions muddle your thinking. Nevertheless, I began to pick up my records monthly.

I soon realized the information was riddled with errors, and I was being given medication for health issues I did not have. *The hospital records listed that I had tuberculosis ... I never had it!*

True or not, it became part of my permanent file. I strongly suggest you get copies of and read your files, so you can promptly correct any errors.

From that point on, I continued to retrieve my records every month and compare them to my own notes from the ER visit or admission. It was disconcerting to find out many things did not match. Many of the records of my ER visits became part fiction due to the inaccuracy of the information.

I also found out that ER professionals incorrectly noted my answers regarding the level of my pain. I was doubled up in pain and the comment in my file was "slight tenderness." I told them I had been vomiting, and they noted I was nauseated. Many hospital notes did not refer to my prior visits accurately and, according to the hospital records, the current visit had no connection to my history.

October 2011 marked the end of my first year of hell. I did not have health insurance at the start of this hellish spiral and 12 months later, I still did not have any insurance. I started to feel as if the staff looked at me as some homeless person who was wasting their time. During a visit to the ER in October 2011, a doctor who felt I did not need anything spoke abruptly to me, and dismissed me without treatment. I left in tears.

While I agree that doctors have substantially more training than I do, they may not be as experienced as you think. Keep in mind that ER personnel may be rotating through the ER for their first shift ever, and you may be their first ER patient. You deserve to have a doctor who will look at you as an individual and treat your symptoms as such. You need a doctor who will investigate the root cause, and not merely look at your symptoms.

People have their own genetic make-ups. Your body chemistry may be different from that of others.

You may exhibit similar symptoms, but you could have a more urgent health need than in more typical cases.

My sixth, seventh, eighth, ninth, and tenth diagnoses: SIBO, leaky gut syndrome, telescoping intestine, ulcerative colitis, and Cohn's disease

Months went by in 2012 and I was still in a state of depression, as well as in constant pain. I had become reluctant to go to the ER for help, but during this year, doctors nonetheless diagnosed me several more times.

### SIBO

SIBO is an acronym for small intestinal bacterial overgrowth syndrome.

It is common with IBS, and with digestive problems involving bloat, gas, abdominal pain, diarrhea, and constipation caused by fermenting of carbohydrates (starches and sugars). In addition, SIBO is often associated with leaky gut syndrome, (which will be discussed in the next section.) (5) (6)

## Symptoms of SIBO:

- bloating
- abdominal pain
- nausea
- diarrhea

Dr. Allison Siebecker (7)states, "The main symptoms of SIBO are those of irritable bowel syndrome (IBS). SIBO has been shown to exist in up to 84% of IBS patients." (7)

### Leaky Gut Syndrome

Leaky gut syndrome occurs when tiny gaps in the membrane lining of your intestinal tract allow large undigested food particles into your bloodstream, causing systemic symptoms such as skin rash, headaches, joint pain, autoimmune disorders, etc. These food particles are toxic substances, which should be confined to your digestive tract, but escape into your bloodstream, hence the term leaky gut syndrome. Leaky gut syndrome is a common cause of food intolerance. This condition can cause you to pack on the pounds, and causes symptoms very similar to those of SIBO. (8)

## Possible Symptoms of Leaky Gut Syndrome:

- bloating
- pain
- unexplained ailments of the intestine

Our small intestine, which is responsible for about 70% of our immune system, behaves like a selective sieve. It lets only nutrients and well-digested fats, proteins, and starches enter the bloodstream and keeps out large molecules, microbes, and toxins.

### Telescoping Intestine

The shape of our intestine is like a long tube. Intussusceptions occur when one part of your intestine, usually the small intestine, slides inside an adjacent part. Sometimes this is also called *telescoping*, because it is similar to the way a collapsible telescope folds together.

Because intussusception is rare in adults, and symptoms of the disorder are often nonspecific, it is more challenging to identify. (9)

## Symptoms of a Telescoping Intestine:

- abdominal pain
- nausea
- vomiting and diarrhea

The doctors considered ulcerative colitis and Crohn's disease, two additional possible diagnoses. Inflammatory bowel disease (IBD) is a general term that includes two main disorders: ulcerative colitis and Crohn's disease.

These two diseases are related, but they are considered separate disorders with somewhat different treatment options. The basic distinctions are location and severity.

Approximately 10% of patients with early stages of IBD have features and symptoms that match the criteria for both ulcerative colitis and Crohn's disease. This is called indeterminate colitis. (10)

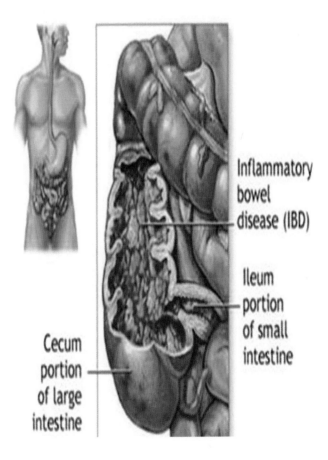

Inflammatory bowel disease (IBD)

Ileum portion of small intestine

Cecum portion of large intestine

Symptoms for *Ulcerative Colitis*

- abdominal Pain
- diarrhea
- bloating
- nausea

Symptoms *Crohn's Disease*

- abdominal Pain
- diarrhea
- bloating
- nausea

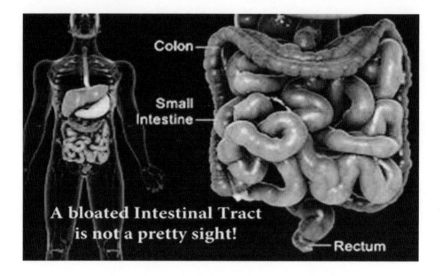

As they say, one picture is worth a thousand words.

Now you know how I felt!

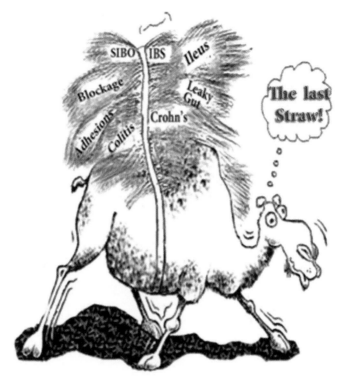

March 2012 was the breaking Point

In March of 2012, I was in horrific pain and cried through the night, but would not allow my husband to take me to the emergency room. My husband was beside himself and told me he was taking me, and that was final. My hesitation in going to the ER was because my relationship with the ER staff had gone steadily downhill since April Fool's day of 2011. I did not have much faith in them, and they were not sure if I was crazy or had a drug addiction.

I delayed him as long as I could, but the pain got to the point where I gave in, and he took me to the hospital.

Up to this point, I had been in the ER approximately 39 times with five admissions.

This particular time I had an ER doctor who had seen me before, and was abrupt with me in the past but this time he humiliated me to the breaking point.

He told me that I had been given a million dollar work up and nothing was wrong with me. He said he had almost lost his license because of another patient who wanted pain medication, and he was not giving me anything. He finished by saying, "I am not going to waste any more resources on tests. You have had too much exposure to radiation, and I'm not putting my job on the line for someone that is not ill."

When I reached home that day, I was in the worst place mentally and physically that I had ever experienced. I was so mentally, emotionally, and physically lost I had no idea what to do next.

I could not keep my mind from racing. I could not complete a sentence, or remember things that had just happened. I could not sleep, and I was frightened. I knew that my brain was not producing the serotonin it needed to provide me with a sense of well being. It was largely due to my medication, but the reason did not matter. It was quite a flip for me. I had gone from being energetic and goal oriented to being stagnant.

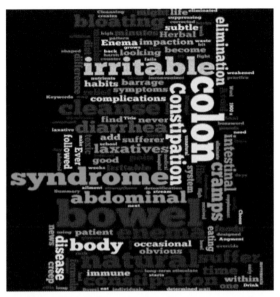

Eventually, it all boiled down to the doctors providing me with a final catchall diagnosis of irritable bowel syndrome (IBS).

After two and a half years of pure hell, I was told I had a non-specific diagnosis. Once again, I had a new starting point. I was hoping this time they finally got it right.

Irritable Bowel Syndrome (IBS) (11) Irritable bowel syndrome (IBS) is a common disorder that affects your large intestine (colon).

Symptoms of IBS:

- cramping
- abdominal pain
- bloating
- pain
- gas
- diarrhea and /or constipation
- flatulence

Despite these uncomfortable signs and symptoms, IBS does not cause permanent damage to your colon. Most people with IBS find that symptoms improve as they learn to control their condition. Only a small number of people with irritable bowel syndrome have disabling signs and symptoms.

Unlike intestinal diseases which are more serious, such as ulcerative colitis and Crohn's disease, irritable bowel syndrome is not apparent on x-rays or scans, does not demonstrate inflammation or changes in bowel tissue, nor does it increase your risk of colorectal cancer. It can also be defined as a functional gastrointestinal disorder, which causes abdominal pain with some alteration of bowel habit.

Some people can have a form of IBS called "diarrhea predominant," which causes abdominal pain. Often you might get the pain after a meal, or when under stress. Based on the criteria, the pain could be relieved after a bowel movement. This was not the case for me. The pain continued no matter what.

I found the information beneficial, but I asked one question. If IBS does not demonstrate inflammation or changes apparent on a scan, then what were the shadows and images the doctors saw that prompted them to diagnosis me with ten other GI disorders?

Was it possible that in essence after all these months, my doctors really had no idea what was wrong with me? My diagnosis was now irritable bowel syndrome, yet they continued to treat my symptoms with multiple medications.

After all my research, I have come to a conclusion in regards to this diagnosis. I share a belief with thousands of individuals, that IBS is not an illness it is a list of symptoms and it is the dumping ground for patients when their doctors can't figure out what is wrong. Hell they had to call it something. I don't think telling a patient that you have, "I don't have a flipping clue disease" will garner much support.

Therefore, my final diagnosis was irritable bowel syndrome (IBS). My gastroenterologist told me nothing could be done but to treat the symptoms. He said they would try to control my IBS with painkillers, anti-diarrhea medication or laxatives, antispasmodics, anti-flatulents, steroids, and other medications.

In short, this meant that the quality of my life was never going to improve. I found a future of taking these drugs incomprehensible. I was not willing to compromise my quality of life.

My local specialist realized how frustrated I was, and he recommended I go to a specialist at a research hospital. He mentioned two or three research hospitals where perhaps they could shed more light on my illness. Perhaps this was the turning point I needed. Would these research hospitals be the light at the end of the tunnel I desperately sought, or empty hope?

Each of the eleven diagnoses had been given had very similar if not exact symptoms but I found only one common element that exacerbated all of the illnesses!

*Areas that should have been researched and weren't—was/is the Vagus Nerve and Mesenteric Vein/*

## VAGUS NERVE AND MESENTERIC VEIN

THEIR IMPACT ON OUR INTESTINAL ILLNESSES!

## Vasovagal Reflex

Why do some IBS sufferers have these symptoms? The most likely explanation is the body's own vasovagal reflex.

The reflex stems from our VAGUS NERVE, which is a nerve that travels from our brains to our COLON and contributes to a wide variety of physical functions, including swallowing, speaking, heart rate and digestion.

The vasovagal reflex is a sudden triggering of the vagus nerve. This may occur in response to a variety of factors, including:

- Fear
- Emotional stress
- Gastrointestinal illness

The following symptoms may occur during a meal or 15-30 minutes following a meal.

- Bloating
- Belching
- Nausea
- Abdominal pain, cramps
- Diarrhea
- Dizziness, lightheadedness

When symptoms develop1-3 hours after eating they may include:

- Weakness, fatigue
- Low blood sugar
- Sweating
- Diarrhea
- Shakiness
- Anxiety
- Heart palpitations
- Fainting
- Mental confusion

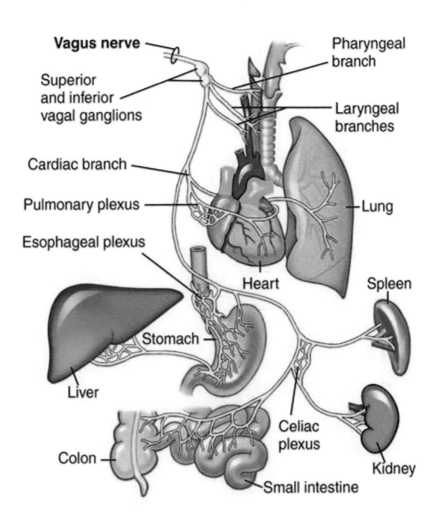

**Vagus nerve**

Superior and inferior vagal ganglions

Cardiac branch

Pulmonary plexus

Esophageal plexus

Pharyngeal branch

Laryngeal branches

Lung

Heart

Spleen

Liver

Stomach

Colon

Celiac plexus

Kidney

Small intestine

## Symptoms of Mesenteric Vein

Early signs and symptoms of acute mesenteric ischemia include:

- Severe abdominal pain, concentrated in one area of the abdomen
- Nausea and/or vomiting
- Bloody stools
- History of chronic atrial fibrillation or cardiovascular disease

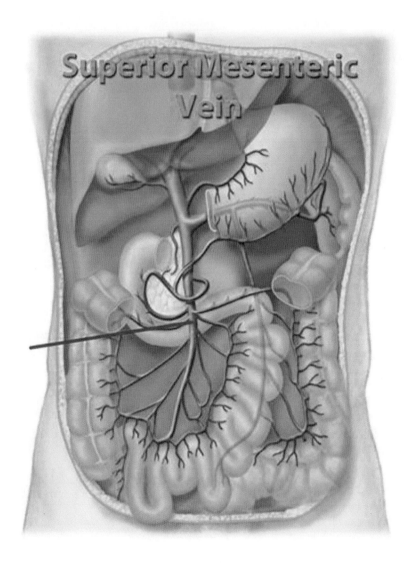

What are intestinal ischemic syndromes?

Intestinal ischemic syndromes -- also called visceral or mesenteric ischemic syndromes -- occur when blood flow to the bowel or gastrointestinal system (intestines) is decreased because of a blood vessel blockage.

The three major abdominal blood vessels that may become blocked include the celiac artery, superior mesenteric artery or inferior mesenteric artery. Usually two or three of these arteries must be narrowed or blocked to cause intestinal ischemic syndromes.

What causes these syndromes?

In most cases, intestinal ischemic syndromes are caused by atherosclerosis (buildup of fatty matter and plaque on the blood vessel walls), leading to narrowing or blockage of the vessel. The conditions also can be caused by blood clots or aneurysms (an abnormal enlargement or bulging) in the vessels.

Are these conditions more common at a certain age?

Intestinal ischemic syndromes are more common after age 60 but can occur at any age.

Types of Intestinal Ischemic Syndromes

Intestinal ischemic syndromes can occur suddenly (acute) or over time (chronic).

Acute Mesenteric Ischemia: The arteries supplying oxygen-rich blood and nutrients to your intestines can become narrowed from atherosclerosis in the same way that coronary (heart) arteries become narrowed in heart disease. Mesenteric ischemia can develop if the narrowing or blockage become severe.

The organs of the gastrointestinal system are responsible for the digestion of food.

Therefore, decreased blood supply to these organs cause symptoms related to eating or after-meal digestion, including:

- Abdominal pain after meals
- Weight loss
- Fear of eating or change in eating habits due to post-meal pain
- Nausea and/or vomiting
- Constipation or diarrhea
- History of cardiovascular disease (such as peripheral arterial disease, stroke, coronary artery disease or heart attack)

| Outcomes of acute mesenteric ischemia | | | |
|---|---|---|---|
| Variable | Endovascular (n = 56) | Surgery (n = 14) | P |
| Complications (%) | | | |
| • Acute renal failure | 27 | 50 | .14 |
| • Pulmonary failure | 27 | 64 | <.05 |
| • Myocardial infarction | 2 | 0 | .99 |
| • Gastrointestinal bleeding | 7 | 14 | .68 |
| • Access-site bleeding | 9 | n/a | n/a |
| • Stroke | 2 | 14 | .12 |
| Mortality (%) | 39 | 50 | .15 |
| • Endovascular success | 36 | n/a | <.05* |
| • Endovascular failures | 50 | n/a | .92* |

\* Compared with mortality of surgery

Arthurs ZM, Titus J, Bannazadeh M, Eagleton MJ, Srivastava S, Sarac TP, Clair DG. A comparison of endovascular revascularization with traditional therapy for the treatment of acute mesenteric ischemia. J Vasc Surg. 2011 Jan 12 [Epub ahead of print]

### Early Pain Theories and Remedies

Since ancient times, humans have sought to conquer pain using a variety of treatments ranging from the sublime to the bizarre. The Greeks and Romans were the first to advance a theory of sensation, the idea that the brain and nervous system have a role in producing the perception of pain. However, it was not until the Middle Ages and well into the Renaissance—the 1400s and 1500s—that evidence began to accumulate in support of these theories.

In the seventeenth and eighteenth centuries, the study of the body—and the senses—continued. In 1664 the French philosopher René Descartes described what, to this day, is still called a *pain pathway.* In the nineteenth century, the application of new chemical and scientific techniques led to the development of morphine, codeine, and heroin—potent pain medications derived from opium. Another potent pain medication and appetite suppressant—cocaine—was successfully isolated from coca leaves by a German chemist during this time. The isolation of these drugs and their subsequent availability in tablet and powder forms led to their widespread adoption as pain medications.

In 1899, aspirin was isolated from salicylate-rich plants. The development of "pure" aspirin was a major breakthrough in the history of pain medications. To this day aspirin is the most commonly used pain reliever worldwide.

### Unrelieved Pain Has Consequences—There Are Many Adverse Effects of Unrequited Acute Pain

It turns out that healing is actually delayed when pain caused by tissue damage is not relieved.

Research shows that uncontrolled pain has an adverse effect on our immune system. Continuous pain also appears to lower our body's ability to respond to stressful situations such as surgery, chemotherapy, and psychological stress.

Far-reaching consequences can also result from pain due to damage to a nerve (neuropathic pain). This type of unrelieved pain seems to cause changes in the nervous system that contribute to the development of chronic pain long after the damage to the nerve has healed.

We already know that controlling pain helps to provide enjoyment and peace to those who are living with a life-threatening illness, but pain control may also prolong life by reducing the negative effects that pain has on the body.

Pain is a fundamentally noxious sensation. Unrelieved acute pain has adverse physical, psychological and economic consequences. It causes voluntary or involuntary splinting of respiratory muscles resulting in pooling of secretions, promoting the development of pneumonia, atelectasis, and ventilation-perfusion abnormalities. Increased serum levels of neuroendocrine hormones cause hyperalgesia, promote glycogenolysis, oxidation of free fatty acids, protein catabolism, sodium and water retention and kaliuresis (causing hypertension, tachycardia and aggravating congestive heart failure), and modify coagulation and fibrinolytic activity. [10,11]

Pain and anxiety also cause anorexia, insomnia, depression and feelings of hopelessness and helplessness. This combination of pain and emotional stress is termed suffering. Perception of pain by the patient may be higher if subjected to the same noxious stimulus the second time around.[12] Unrelieved pain results in longer hospital stays, increased rate of re-hospitalization, increased outpatient visits and decreased level of function, leading to loss of income and insurance coverage.[13]

Persistent Pain is a Debilitating Presence That Affects a Patient's Ability to Perform Normal Activities of Daily Living.

The consequences of chronic pain are far-reaching and go beyond physical sensations of ongoing discomfort. Research shows that unrelieved pain negatively affects patients in every way – socially, physically and financially.

According to a review by researchers from the National Center for Complementary and Alternative Medicine, published in Nature Reviews Neuroscience in 2013, chronic pain can alter brain circuitry and lead to a faster loss of gray matter, increase sensitivity to pain signals, reduce ability of the brain to release its own painkillers and cause emotional changes (such as anxiety disorders and depression) and cognitive deficits. Chronic pain can lead to medical problems that can result in immobility, malnutrition and an increased risk of falling.

History of "Oligoanalgesia"

Wilson and Pendleton coined the word "oligoanalgesia," to represent the failure to recognize or properly treat pain.[5] Sir. Zachary Cope, one of the doyens of surgery, in his book Early Diagnosis of the Acute Abdomen suggested "Though it may appear cruel, it is really kind to withhold morphine until one is certain or not that surgical interference is necessary, i.e. until a reasonable diagnosis has been made."[6] This sentiment has pervaded medical practice until recent times.

Historically, and to some extent today, abdominal pain is a clinical diagnosis; a definite cause is often obscure in over 40 percent of cases.[7] Analgesics were thought to hinder the ability to reach a diagnosis, leading to large numbers of negative work-ups and unnecessary surgeries.

Withholding analgesics was thought to minimize the increased burden on patient and hospital resources, resulting from delay in diagnosis and inappropriate treatment.

As recently as 1996, a majority of surgeons considered that analgesics interfered with patient's signing a valid informed consent and impacted diagnostic accuracy, thus influencing their decision to withhold pain relief.[8]

The attitudes regarding treatment of pain are shifting, nevertheless slowly. A prospective study of 100 emergency admissions for acute abdominal pain by Tait et al showed that most of the trained surgical staff (88%) favored early administration of analgesia in the ED and a majority (79%) would administer analgesia in the absence of a firm diagnosis.[9]

The Tait study, however, also showed that the mean "door to analgesia" time in the ED was 2.3 hours for patients with severe pain and 6.3 hours for moderate pain, even though all patients were assessed almost immediately (within 20 minutes) by a trainee physician. Nearly half of the patients in the study were transferred to the floor without analgesia having been given (mean wait 5.7 hours).[9]

Clinical diagnosis did not influence the speed or urgency with which patients received analgesia. In the study, almost half the surgical trainees believed that analgesics would mask the diagnostic features and delay appropriate management. This discrepancy between the opinions of the surgeons and the trainees explained the discordance between surgical staff sentiment and actual practice.[9]

The Importance of Pain Control

Although pain can protect us by forcing us to rest an injury or to stop doing something, the experience of being in a state of uncontrolled pain is horrible, frightening, and can have a profound effect on our quality of life.

Uncontrolled pain can:

- delay healing
- decrease appetite
- increase stress
- disrupt sleep
- cause anxiety and depression

## Understanding Pain—Gate Theory of Pain

Due to the observations that raised questions, a new theory of pain was developed in the early 1960s to account for the clinically recognized importance of the mind and brain in pain perception. It is called the *gate control theory of pain*, and it was initially developed by Ronald Melzack and Patrick Wall.

Although the theory accounts for phenomena that are primarily mental in nature - that is, pain itself as well as some of the psychological factors influencing it - its scientific beauty is that it provides a physiological basis for the complex phenomenon of pain.

It does this by investigating the complex structure of the nervous system, which is comprised of the following two major divisions:

- Central nervous system (the spinal cord and the brain)
- Peripheral nervous system (nerves outside of the brain and spinal cord, including branching nerves in the torso and extremities, as well as nerves in the lumbar spine region)

In the gate control theory, the experience of pain depends on a complex interplay of these two systems as they each process pain signals in their own way. Upon injury, pain messages originate in nerves associated with the damaged tissue and flow along the peripheral nerves to the spinal cord and on up to the brain. So far, this is roughly equivalent to the specificity theory of pain described above.

However, in the gate control theory, before they can reach the brain these pain messages encounter "nerve gates" in the spinal cord that open or close depending upon a number of factors (possibly including instructions coming down from the brain). When the gates are opening, pain messages "get through" more or less easily and pain can be intense. When the gates close, pain messages are prevented from reaching the brain and may not even be experienced.

Although no one yet understands the details of this process or how to control it, the following concepts are presented to help explain why various treatments are effective and how to find solutions to chronic back pain.

## The Peripheral Nervous System

Sensory nerves bring information about pain, heat, cold and other sensory phenomena to the spinal cord from various parts of the body. At least two types of nerve fibers are thought to carry the majority of pain messages to the spinal cord:

- A-delta nerve fibers, which carry electrical messages to the spinal cord at approximately 40 mph ("first" or "fast" pain).
- C-fibers, which carry electrical messages at approximately 3 mph to the spinal cord ("slow" or "continuous pain")

A good example of how these respective nerve fibers work is the activation of the A-delta nerve fibers followed by the activation of the slower C-fibers. The activation of other types of nerve fibers can modify or block the sensation of pain.

After hitting one's elbow or head, rubbing the area seems to provide some relief. This activates other sensory nerve fibers that are even "faster" than A-delta fibers, and these fibers send information about pressure and touch that reach the spinal cord and brain to override some of the pain messages carried by the A-delta and C-fibers.

I was going through some of my research and I found several articles on breaking the Pain Cycle.

If you have had any of the "Invisible Illnesses", you will realize the only thing that is "Invisible" is finding a doctor who can find the "Root" of each patient's complaints. I have read and heard repeatedly that that the patient is made to feel that their health issues are in their heads.

I was in the hospital recently and I overheard a patient pleading with the Doctor that his health issues are not in his head—he is really in pain and no one seems to be listening. Often the medical professionals make us (the patients) feel it is in our head due to their lack of knowledge to the issue at hand. I wanted to reach over and grab the curtain and let them know "I know it is not in your head!" The patient's immediate concern was that the medical professional was going to tell him that it was "in his head". This happens so frequently that I have even met with the ER Physician of the hospital I go to in order to get them on the same page as their patient.

The pain is very real but can be the result of an interaction between the Gut and Brain.

I've had discussed the brain—gut relationship in the past and how, in many cases a downward pain cycle involving the mind and Gut leads to increasing pain levels, as well as emotional distress.

Short definition is "Pain makes you Tense" and "Tension increases your Pain!"

Stress Pain Cycle

A normal physical response to stress is to tighten the muscles in our shoulders, jaw, fists and other areas. If you already have pain in these areas, tightening the muscles can lead to increased pain.

Even if you don't have pain, staying in a prolonged state of muscle tension due to stress can lead to restricted blood flow to the muscles, eventually leading to pain. In both cases, if you don't address the 'mind' part, the pain will likely continue and may even worsen.

In addition to muscle tension, stress results in hormonal and neurotransmitter changes in the body, which can contribute to pain. These changes involve biochemicals such as serotonin, cortisol, endorphins, norepinephrine and dopamine. We will revisit all of these in more detail in future posts, but for now let us briefly look at the stress hormone, cortisol.

Cortisol is called the "stress hormone" because it is a key hormone involved in our stress response. Under short-term stress, cortisol is beneficial and is associated with reduced sensation of pain and improved healing. Under long-term stress, however, abnormal patterns of cortisol secretion can occur affecting the immune system, resulting in inflammation and autoimmune disorders. This in turn, can lead to increased pain and slowed healing.

"Pain makes you Tense" and "Tension increases your Pain!"

Now for the vicious cycle. As many of you may know, having chronic pain can be intensely stressful due to not only the pain, but also the loss of activity, relationships, job, finances and hobbies. When feeling the stress from the pain, you may tighten your muscles without even knowing it and your biochemistry may be in stress mode. As a result, you may feel more pain that then leads to even more stress, resulting in a downward pain cycle from which it is hard to break out.

If or when I have a flare-up, I place myself on semi-bowel rest for one to two days—water and 4 ounces of protein is all I will eat during my semi-bowel rest. I lay completely flat and concentrate on relaxing. Your pain will not improve if you don't learn how to relax and what works for you.

See more at: http://www.whatworksforpain.com/2010/02/stress-pain-cycle-part-i-of-the-downward-cycle-of-chronic-pain/#sthash.sh3Kdwyw.dpuf

Debunking Pain Myths

Sometimes, misconceptions about pain can get in the way of pain control. Here are some common misunderstandings about pain.

- Pain happens; you just need to put up with it.
    - o Pain control and comfort is a reasonable expectation. Pain does not have to be tolerated, but can be treated to improve your comfort and quality of life.
- If I take pain medication too early, it won't work when the pain gets really bad.
    - o When treated early, pain is easier to control. There are many options for controlling pain.
- I will get addicted to narcotic pain medications.
    - o The majority of people taking opioid (narcotic) pain medications for pain do not become addicted. Some people will develop tolerance (need higher doses of the medication over time) or physical dependence (experience withdrawal symptoms if the medication is stopped suddenly), but these can be managed.
- Doctor and nurses are so busy. I don't want to bother them.
    - o Yes, nurses and doctors are busy, but you have the right to have your pain controlled and they don't want to see you in pain.
    - o Even if they seem too busy, it's important to let your nurse or doctor know when your pain is not controlled.

Before discussing the details of pain control, it is important to understand that having trust in your health care team is essential for good pain management. To establish this trust, you need those around you, especially your health care team, to believe that your pain is what you say it is. This is the key that will allow you and your health care team to work together to help you deal with the pain.

In addition, it is very helpful to get an explanation for the pain - what is causing it and why it is occurring. The unknown pain always hurts more than the known pain. Indeed, knowing the source of the pain is one of the first steps to being able to control it.

Being able to talk about the pain will also help you to cope better—how it affects you and how you feel about what is causing it. As well, it is crucial to be able to discuss other issues in your life, either with the people around you or a member of your health care team. If you are worried about relationships, spiritual issues, your future health, finances, or other issues, your pain will be magnified.

Today there are many options available to adequately control pain, and pain control is something you can aim for. You may have to balance the level of pain control with certain medication side effects, but pain control should be your goal.

## The Costs of Pain

The 6 million Canadians who live with pain carry a unique bundle of burdens. Beyond the actual physical sensation of pain, the costs of pain can be far-reaching and life changing, affecting the day-to-day life of the one in pain and those close to them in many unexpected and challenging ways.

For those living with it, pain can be devastating and disruptive to the flow of life. With pain, you may feel unable to go to work, to interact with friends and family, or to do your usual daily life activities.

Pain can interfere with sleep and affect your mood. This loss of ability and independence can, in turn, affect your sense of self-worth and self-esteem.

The cold, hard fact is that pain affects a person's quality of life in significant ways. In fact, compared to people living with other chronic diseases, those with chronic pain have a lower quality of life and a higher risk of suicide.

Because pain is not visible like a rash or sudden like a heart attack, a person with pain may be doubted by doctors, co-workers, employers, and even by friends and family.

## The Impact of Pain on Friends and Family

Pain burdens the person feeling the pain, but it can also weigh on those around them in many ways.

Family and friends experience the emotional stress of seeing someone they care about dealing with pain. This can lead to feelings of sadness - imagine the sting of no longer being able to hold or carry your children. Alternatively, this lead to feelings of anger or resentment for the effort and attention that must be given to the person in pain.

Relatives often become caregivers, sacrificing their own time and energy to attend to tasks that have become difficult for the one in pain. Household members may see roles and responsibilities switch to accommodate the needs of the one in pain. Moreover, the financial burden of pain - health care costs, lost workdays - can become a point of intense stress in a family.

Many with moderate to severe chronic pain are forced to cut back on work hours, reduce responsibilities, lose income, or even abandon their jobs completely. In addition, a person living with pain will likely not only lose income - they will also gain expenses from treatments and medications.

In broader terms, pain comes with a very high price tag. The cost of chronic pain is estimated at more than $10 billion each year. This includes the costs of lost income, lost productivity, and the expenses of medical treatments.

## Abstract

Acute abdominal pain is one of the most common chief complaints of patients presenting to emergency departments. Historically, physicians have been reluctant to treat this pain with analgesics because of fear of obscuring physical findings, which were often critical to proper diagnosis and treatment

Methods: Articles highlighting the role of analgesics in acute abdominal pain were reviewed, with particular emphasis on the practice of Oligoanalgesia (undertreating pain), effects of unrelieved pain, the beneficial or detrimental effects of analgesics, and methods of analgesic administration.

Results and conclusions: Studies indicate that unrelieved pain has serious adverse physiologic, psychologic and economic consequences. Providing immediate pain relief after stabilizing patients may not affect diagnostic ability or subsequent surgical decision-making capacity, and indeed may be beneficial in making a diagnosis.

Many practical suggestions exist for how to best provide analgesia in abdominal pain.

Given this evidence, appropriate and aggressive treatment resulting in prompt relief of acute abdominal pain is the desirable standard of care. A protocol to alert other involved physicians of analgesic administration is important.

## Emergency Room and your Gut

Acute abdominal pain is one of the most common chief patient complaints in emergency departments (ED), and constitutes 6.4% of the 100 million ED patient visits each year.[1,2] Twenty five percent of general surgical admissions present primarily with acute abdominal pain.[3] In 25 percent of patients presenting with pain to the ED as the chief complaint, the pain is abdominal.[4] In many acute care settings, analgesics are often withheld in patients with acute abdominal pain for fear that it may change physical examination findings, delaying diagnosis and treatment.

The medical community's interest and understanding of pain is evolving and to many, it is now the fifth vital sign. Advances in the management of chronic pain and end-of-life issues have also focused attention on the adverse effects of unrelieved pain.

The reason I added this to my post today is to encourage you—to explore the historical reasons for withholding analgesia, the drawbacks of this strategy, the evidence for a new paradigm and some practical tools to help in providing analgesia for acute abdominal pain.

## Principles of Pain Assessment and Causes of Under-Treatment of Acute Pain

The patient's self-report is the most reliable indicator of the presence and intensity of pain. Physicians should trust patient's subjective reports of pain unless there is evidence to the contrary.

Age, sex, ethnicity, and cognitive functioning of the patient influence the assessment and treatment of pain.[26,27,28,29,30,31,32] Children, the elderly, the cognitively impaired, and those with communication problems are often more difficult to assess and require special attention to ensure adequacy of analgesia. Pain assessment tools (eg. A visual analog scale) should be available in the ED and should be utilized appropriately.

The degree of pain, the suspected underlying pathology, pain response to titration of the drug, and side effects should determine the analgesic, dosing and frequency of use.

The principles of the "analgesic ladder" (non-opioid analgesics for mild to moderate pain, oral opioids- oxycodone for moderate to severe pain and parenteral opioids for severe pain), may be used to guide the choice of the analgesic.[33]

Some barriers to effective pain management include reluctance on the part of patients to report pain or use analgesics, state and federal policies regarding the use of opioid analgesics, limited provider knowledge about pain assessment and treatment, and underuse of analgesics because of provider misconceptions regarding addiction.[34,35,36] Under-treatment may also arise from failure to inquire about pain, discrediting reports of pain (pain judged to be less than reported), and educational or psychological barriers on the part of the physician.[37,38,39,40]

Pseudo addiction (inadequate pain management producing the manipulative behavior on the part of the patient) may be much more common than addiction. A retrospective review of over 12,000 hospitalized patients given opioids for pain relief identified only four who were potential addicts.[41] Alcohol abuse or drug addiction does not interfere with a patient's ability to identify painful stimuli and should not bar providing adequate pain relief; these patients may benefit from carefully supervised, judicious use of analgesics.

70

Tolerance may also dictate a greater frequency in analgesic use, though true pharmacological tolerance requiring escalating analgesic doses is uncommon.[42] (12)


Chronic Pain Fact Sheet/by Marcia E. Bedard, PhD


In past months, a growing amount of media attention has been given to the unspeakable suffering of millions of Americans with incurable conditions causing severe chronic pain. In addition to articles in the popular press and segments on network television, the Internet is an increasingly rich source of information on this topic. Yet the agonizing pain of millions of chronic pain patients remains untreated. This is largely because the nation's War on Drugs has created a climate of fear among patients and health professionals alike — fears of using strong opioid medications, which are often the only way to relieve severe pain when all other treatments have failed.

This fact sheet is intended to debunk some of the myths that fuel this unreasonable fear, and is being sent to legislators, patients, and health professionals throughout the nation. It will also enable members of the press to have quick access to credible facts about chronic pain. Although this fact sheet shows the devastating effects on physical and mental health when severe pain goes untreated, as well as the profound impact on the economy, there is no way to measure the "bankruptcies of the heart" that invariably accompany this condition. Yet the steady erosion of the quality of life for millions of pain patients and their families — as they struggle with divorce, poverty, homelessness, despair, and often suicide — is the real tragedy here.

FACT SHEET ON CHRONIC NONMALIGNANT PAIN (CNP)

CNP, pain that lasts six months or more and does not respond well to conventional medical treatment, affects more people than any other type of pain.

Thirty-four million Americans suffer from chronic pain, and most are significantly disabled by it, sometimes permanently. [1, 2, 15]

The economic impact of CNP is staggering. Back pain, migraines, and arthritis alone account for medical costs of $40 billion annually, and pain is the cause of 25% of all sick days taken yearly. The annual total cost of pain from all causes is estimated to be more than $100 billion. [2, 4, 15]

Despite the magnitude of suffering, CNP remains grossly undertreated in most patients. The reasons for this are: the low priority of pain relief in our health care system; lack of knowledge among both health professionals and consumers about pain management; exaggerated fears of opioid side effects and addiction; and health professionals' fear of medical board and DEA scrutiny, even when controlled substances are used appropriately for pain relief. [2, 13, 14, 15]

Contrary to common fears, numerous studies have shown addiction is extremely rare in pain patients taking opioid drugs, even in patients with histories of drug abuse and/or addiction.

CNP patients will develop a physical dependence on opioid drugs, but this is not the same thing as addiction, which is an aberrant psychological state. [2, 3, 4, 5, 6, 7, 8, 9, 10, 11, 13, 14]

- Unrelieved pain has many negative health consequences including, but not limited to: increased stress, metabolic rate, blood clotting and water retention; delayed healing; hormonal imbalances; impaired immune system and gastrointestinal functioning; decreased mobility; problems with appetite and sleep, and needless suffering. CNP also causes many psychological problems, such as feelings of low self-esteem, powerlessness, hopelessness, and depression. [12, 15, 16, 18, 19]

- Under treatment of CNP often results in suicide. In a recent survey, 50% of CNP patients had inadequate pain relief and had considered suicide to escape the unrelenting agony of their pain. Unrelieved pain also leads to requests for physician-assisted suicide, another indicator of pain's harsh impact on the quality of life of many patients and their families. [7, 8, 13, 14, 15, 16]

- Discrimination against CNP patients is pervasive in the American health care system. Women, racial/ethnic minorities, children, the elderly, worker's compensation patients, and previously disabled patients (e.g., those with cerebral palsy, or who are deaf, blind, amputees, survivors of childhood polio, etc.) are at great risk for under treatment of their pain, even though patients belonging to one or more of these groups are the vast majority of all CNP patients. [2, 13, 17]

- CNP patients with severe, unrelenting pain from permanent structural damage to the neurologic or musculo-skeletal systems are often subjected to expensive and unnecessary surgeries and other painful invasive procedures. Arachnoiditis and reflex sympathetic dystrophy are the most common causes of severe CNP. Other common causes include post-trauma, adhesions, systemic lupus, headaches, degenerative arthritis, fibromyalgia, and neuropathies. [8, 15, 18, 19] (13)References Page Source Documents 307

## Pain Often Undertreated

Despite the billions of dollars spent to treat pain, it is often inadequately treated, particularly in vulnerable populations such as children, older adults, and ethnic minorities. Patients with cognitive impairments, cancer patients, and those with active addiction or a history of substance abuse are also often undertreated. Add to this the many people who lack a usual source of care, low level of trust in clinicians, low expectation of treatment outcomes, language barrier, and communication difficulty (IOM, 2011) and a bleak picture emerges.

Somewhat surprisingly, under-treatment of pain can even be an issue for patients with diseases known to cause pain, such as cancer, HIV/AIDS, and sickle-cell anemia. In a study of 1,308 outpatients with metastatic cancer from 54 cancer treatment centers:

- 62% had pain severe enough to impair their ability to function

- 42% reported they were not given adequate analgesic therapy (AHRQ, 2008)

Many studies have reported that all classes of analgesic, particularly opioid analgesics, are under-utilized in the treatment of pain associated with AIDS (Fishman et al., 2010). One study noted that about half of respondents said they could not afford the prescribed analgesic, had no access to a pain specialist, or were reluctant to take opioids out of concern that others will think they are abusing pain medications (Fishman et al., 2010). HIV-infected women with pain were twice as likely to be under-treated as their male counterparts (Lohman et al., 2010)

In a survey of 500 AIDS care *providers*, primarily physicians and nurses reported:

- Lack of knowledge regarding pain management

- Reluctance to prescribe opioids

- Lack of access to pain specialists

- Concerns about drug abuse or addiction

- Concerns about lack of access to psychological support or drug treatment services (Fishman et al., 2010)

Race and ethnicity are also factors in the under-treatment of pain. In the African American population, lower rates of clinician assessment and higher rates of under-treatment have been found in all settings and across all types of pain (IOM, 2011). Similar results have been found among Hispanics, Asian Americans, and American Indians.

Not surprisingly, nursing home residents do not receive adequate pain control. It's estimated that 45% to 80% of patients in nursing homes have substantial pain that is undertreated.

This suggests that when nursing home residents have moderate to severe pain, they have only about a 50% chance of obtaining adequate pain relief (AHRQ, 2008). (14)

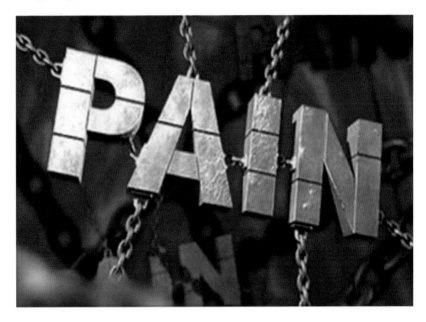

| Illness | Pain Response |
|---|---|
| Cardiovascular | Heart rate, increase cardiac workload, increase peripheral vascular resistance, increase systemic vascular resistance, hypertension, increase coronary vascular resistance, increase myocardial oxygen consumption, hypercoagulation, deep vein thrombosis |
| Cognitive | Muscle spasm, impaired muscle function, fatigue, immobility |
| Developmental | Increase Behavioral and physiologic responses to pain, altered temperaments, higher somatization, infant distress behavior; possible altered development of the pain system, Increase vulnerability to stress disorders, addictive behavior, and anxiety states |
| Future Pain | Debilitating chronic pain syndromes: postmastectomy pain, postthoracotomy pain, phantom pain, postherpetic neuralgia |
| Gastrointestinal | Decreases Gastric and bowel motility |
| Genitourinary | Decrease Urinary output, urinary retention, fluid overload, hypokalemia |
| Immune | Depression of immune response |
| Metabolic | Gluconeogenesis, hepatic glycogenolysis, hyperglycemia, glucose intolerance, insulin resistance, muscle protein catabolism, increase lipolysis |
| Musculoskeletal | Muscle spasm, impaired muscle function, fatigue, immobility |
| Respiratory | decrease Flows and volumes, atelectasis, shunting, hypoxemia, decrease cough, sputum retention, infection |
| Quality of Life | Sleeplessness, anxiety, fear, hopelessness, decrease in sexual desire, Increase thoughts of suicide |

Final Note

Educate yourself of pain, pain management and have an open discussion with your doctor.

I called the recommended research hospitals, they said they would only take me on a cash basis, and the up-front amount ranged from $5,000 to $8,000, which we did not have. With no success with my first two tries, I finally decided to try the doctor in Augusta, Georgia hoping for a better outcome. He was the closest and according to my doctor had an outstanding reputation.

After calling the first two research hospitals I was given, I finally decided to try the doctor in Augusta, Georgia. He was the closest and according to my doctor had an outstanding reputation.

My doctor sent all of my records to the Augusta specialist. I was told that once the doctor looked over my medical records he would decide whether to accept me as a patient.

It just so happened that my medical history matched his current research. He accepted me as a new patient and I was relieved. His office set up appointments and I was scheduled for 3 days of tests. Unfortunately, we were unable to raise the $5,000 needed for the appointment. So no appointment and I felt lost again.

However, I did have the name of the tests that they were going to perform and the name of the doctor who had accepted me as a patient.

With this information in hand, I became driven to find out everything I could in regards to the type of tests they were, as well as the doctor's background. It was during this research, when I happen upon something called fructose malabsorption.

None of the diagnoses I had received was creating my health crisis. No one was able to diagnose me. I found out I lost 2 ½ years of my life to one simple thing: fructose. This word would change my life.

After researching the tests, in addition to the background of the Augusta doctor, I discovered fructose malabsorption/intolerance. Every symptom listed for this illness matched my symptoms from the onset of my health crisis.

My research was in-depth. When I could not get the information I needed from the four well-known respected research hospitals/universities I was working with, I turned to the library, the bookstore, or my own medical reference books.

What I was learning was simple common sense: our bodies have the natural ability to heal themselves. I needed to find out what I could do to help my body to heal. I was desperate to gain additional knowledge to find an answer to my health issues. It wasn't cut and dried but ultimately <u>my own research</u> led to my ACTUAL diagnosis.

## ALL SIMILAR SYMPTOMS, ONE PROBLEM FOR EACH…HFCS!

### Fructose:

Sucrose is table sugar and it's important for you to understand that sucrose breaks down to a fifty-fifty split of glucose and fructose.

As long as the sugar you've eaten has more glucose than fructose, your small intestine should (and I repeat "should") be able to break it down before it reaches your colon (i.e. large intestine). However, there is more to the story.

### Doctors and fructose:

My local doctors knew very little about this issue, but they did know about it.

A simple test could have been given to me very early on and that test would have supported a diagnosis of a form of fructose malabsorption.

Fructose malabsorption (formerly known as dietary fructose intolerance) is not a new issue, but it is an under researched issue.

After months of research, I got myself properly tested and the test results supported my suspicion that I indeed had fructose malabsorption. My issue was, however, more of a problem, because I was finally diagnosed with hereditary fructose intolerance (HFI), which can be life threatening.

As I became educated on the subject of fructose, I realized nothing was going to stop the pain unless I removed this substance from my diet. I thought back to beginning of this nightmare and realized no one ever inquired about my diet ... not one doctor ever asked me what I was eating!

I had been keeping a journal to keep track of all of my health issues, and I highly recommend this practice to anyone who is ill. From such notes a pattern might emerge which could be beneficial in determining a diagnosis.

I thought back to the food I received in the hospital; even the soft foods I was given in during my hospitalizations contained fructose, and that is why my pain continued.

Are irritable bowel syndrome, fructose malabsorption, and hereditary fructose intolerance all connected? In a word: yes! However, there is a more in-depth explanation.

I no longer was the crazy woman who needed attention or the narcotic-addicted drug seeker. Instead, I had an answer … Thank God I had an answer!

## The Final Issue was and is "Fructose!"

From that moment on, this word *fructose* would necessarily begin to dominate my daily thinking. Fructose affects every diagnosis that I have listed. This food additive has become part of our lives, even if most of us didn't even know it existed.

My pain would never go away until the fructose was out of my system!

I had an answer, but now what—where do I from here?

Where was I to go from here? Now that I had a solid starting point, I continued my research in order to have a guide for what to do next.

Nowadays it seems that doctors forget to ask how and why we are suffering maladies. The meaning of the word diagnosis has changed. It no longer means "understand how and why." Instead, it means a word describing a list of symptoms and test results. A code for this word can be entered into a computer; when that code appears, it shows how many days of hospital stay will be approved and what medications are covered by that code. What the doctor thinks really doesn't matter much anymore.

### Finally a Diagnosis and Direction

My twelfth and final diagnosis was hereditary fructose intolerance (HFI).

Although HFI only affects 1 in 20,000 to 30,000 people, fructose malabsorption affects approximately 40% of those individuals who live in the Western hemisphere.

That means, according to the 2012 Census and World Bank, that out of the 313.9 million people in the United States, an approximately 125 and a half million individuals are currently impacted by fructose malabsorption. This may seem a high number to you but many countries will not import our processed-foods so I used just the numbers for country to make this point.

I will provide you with all the information necessary to understand fructose and I will outline for you what you need to do to reclaim your digestive health.

What is Hereditary Fructose Intolerance?

First, hereditary fructose intolerance is rare and can be a life threatening condition.

HFI is severe fructose intolerance due to genetic defects (subnormal activity of aldolase B in the liver, kidney, and small bowel). It is generally diagnosed in young children, but there are many substantiated cases of people reaching age 50 or older before it is diagnosed. HFI and fructose malabsorption have the same symptoms, which present only after the ingestion of fructose. Often HFI goes unchecked in older people because it is unusual and the proper tests are not performed.

In individuals with HFI, fructose creates metabolic disturbances (such as hypoglycemia) and permanent liver and kidney damage can ensue. In infants, HFI may be lethal due to seizures and coma.

After ingesting fructose, individuals with either HFI or fructose, malabsorption may experience nausea, bloating, abdominal pain, diarrhea, vomiting, and low blood sugar (hypoglycemia).

Affected infants may fail to grow and gain weight at the expected rate (failure to thrive).

Hereditary fructose intolerance (HFI) symptoms:

- bloating (from fermentation in the small and large intestine)
- diarrhea and/or constipation
- flatulence
- stomach pain (as a result of muscle spasms…the intensity of which can vary from mild and chronic to acute but erratic)
- nausea
- vomiting (if great quantities are consumed)
- early signs of clinical mental depression
- fuzzy head
- aching eyes
- fatigue
- rapid weight gain or loss
- symptoms of hypoglycemia: sugar craving, tremor, fainting, and in severe cases convulsions or coma.

## Sensitivity

There is even sensitivity to the fructose component of sucrose, household sugar, as well as to infusions containing fructose.

All forms of sucrose and fructose, and probably sorbitol, should be strictly avoided.

A positive family history of sugar intolerance or an aversion against sweets / candies is a useful clue. (I was adopted…so much of my family history was not known.) Diagnosis is by careful history taking, blood sampling for metabolic, liver, and kidney disease, and, specifically, genetic testing. At present, not all forms of HFI can be identified using genetic blood tests. (12)

Since HFI is difficult to diagnose in older people, doctors don't generally perform the tests that are needed to diagnose their patients.

## How Common is HFI?

The incidence of hereditary fructose intolerance is estimated to be 1 in 20,000 to 30,000 individuals each year worldwide.

## What Genes are Related to HFI?

Mutations in the ALDOB gene cause HFI. The ALDOB gene provides instructions for making the aldolase B enzyme. This enzyme is found primarily in the liver and is involved in the breakdown (metabolism) of fructose so this sugar can be used as energy.

Aldolase B is responsible for the second step in the metabolism of fructose, which breaks down the molecule fructose-1-phosphate into other molecules called glyceraldehyde and dihydroxyacetone phosphate.

The death of liver cells and reduced number of phosphate groups lead to hypoglycemia, liver dysfunction, and other features of hereditary fructose intolerance.

Testing...this information, I read in the paper that Dr. Satish Rao Published. He is located in Augusta Georgia and if you have insurance or the cash, Dr. Rao is the person who will help you!

Your Doctor needs to prescribe an HBT test.

The hydrogen breath test (HBT) is used to diagnose intolerance of dietary sugars such as lactose, fructose, or sorbitol. The testing begins by having the patient drink a solution made up of the suspected substance.

If the intolerance exists, the individual does not digest the sugar in the small intestine, so the substance will make its way to the large intestine and be fermented by bacteria in the colon.

The by-product of this fermentation is hydrogen, which is then measured with a breath test administered several hours after the ingestion of the suspected substance.

If no such intolerance exists, the substance is thought to be digested in the small intestine, and there is no rise in breath hydrogen upon testing.

In case of suspicion of severe fructose intolerance in children, a careful history would be taken and specific genetic tests performed to exclude hereditary fructose intolerance (HFI) before performing the fructose breath test. This is recommended to prevent serious reactions to the ingested fructose

There are six types of test to detect if you have a dietary intolerance issue:

- Glucose Breath Test to rule out bacterial overgrowth
- Lactose Breath Test to test for intolerance to milk and milk products
- Fructose Breath Test to determine intolerance to fructose
- Sucrose Breath Test if indicated from physical and oral history
- Stable isotope breath tests for children and pregnant women
- Uric acid blood test

A Georgia specialist, Dr. Satish Rao and his colleagues have worked to standardize the fructose breath test.

They have found a test solution of 25 grams of fructose allows them to identify those people with poor fructose absorption.

It is hard to believe that such a simple test, which can make a huge difference for millions of people, is not readily available.

Part of the problem is many GI doctors are not well informed about the need for breath testing. Further, many GI centers do not have the equipment for conducting breath tests.

This is my advice: while it is valuable to be diagnosed with fructose malabsorption, if that is your ailment, it is more important to take responsibility for your own health and to act now!

There is absolutely no harm in cutting back on your overall fructose intake. Actually, there is a tremendous amount to be gained in terms of better health overall, improved blood-lipid profile, better insulin sensitivity, weight loss, improved blood pressure, and so on.

## How do People Inherit HFI?

This condition is inherited in an autosomal recessive pattern, which means both copies of the gene in each cell have mutations.

The parents of an individual with an autosomal recessive condition each carry one copy of the mutated gene, but they typically do not show signs and symptoms of the condition.

I never experienced any problem until late in life, so if someone tells you that you must not have HFI because you would have had these problems earlier, my experience shows that is not true (in fact, as previously stated, there are many documented cases of the diagnosis being made in individuals that were in their 50's or 60's.)

Remember: hereditary fructose intolerance is a genetic disorder that can be diagnosed at any age.

### Treatment

There is no known pharmaceutical treatment for this health issue the medication you receive is treating the symptoms in hopes of providing relief from pain and discomfort.

### Cure

There is no known cure for malabsorption issues, except to treat the symptoms for relief. Your doctor may prescribe painkillers, anti-diarrheal medication or laxatives, antispasmodic-flatulence medications, or steroids among others.

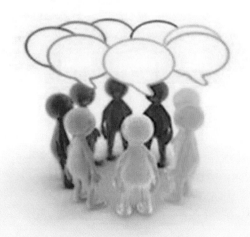

# How did I get this and will my Children or Grandchildren be affected?

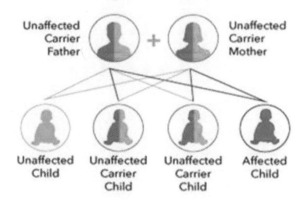

Beware of High Fructose Corn Syrup (HFCS)

Fructose has become even a bigger problem since the end of 1960, primarily due to the invention and use of high fructose corn syrup (HFCS). It could be threatening your digestive health, and therefore your physical and mental well-being. I will delve more into the subject in the following chapters.

# We All Have a Very Strong Connection to Food!

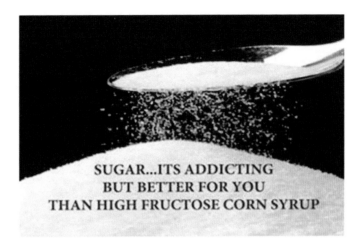

**SUGAR...ITS ADDICTING
BUT BETTER FOR YOU
THAN HIGH FRUCTOSE CORN SYRUP**

So when we hear there must be a change in the types of food we can eat ... it affects us in two major ways.

1. Food is a large part of how we socialize with family and friends
2. Food is tied to many of our memories or events.

Our normal response to anyone even considering changing our eating habits is one of angst. We're all too used to being able to go to the doctor to get a prescription to deal with a health issue. That is not how this works!

Many people go their whole lives plagued by the effects of the many diagnoses I have listed. They never feel completely well, but they assume nothing else can be done.

Moreover, they aren't able to live their lives to the fullest. These individuals have no idea how much better they could feel ... because no one discusses fructose with them.

# Fructose & Your Doctor: You Will Meet With Resistance!

I no longer, personally, have the luxury of wasting another minute of my life with a doctor or any medical professional who can't openly discuss my health and explain my health issues on a level I can understand. If your doctor is not open to a thorough discussion regarding your health then it is time for a change.

A medical professional who understands holistic health as well as the benefits of truly needed pharmaceuticals is the person you need to look for! Many MDs are now prescribing herbs and vitamins that used to be considered an old wives' tale or hogwash.

Food selection, vitamins, herbs, and exercise are being stressed more now than in the past. I am pleased to say the doctors I currently see have included herbs and vitamins as part of my regular treatment regimen.

You should be able to ask questions without being reminded that you are not the doctor in the room. Make sure you ask all the questions you can and demand concise responses to your concerns.

Don't make the assumption that all the tests that can be run have been run. Many times some of the very expensive tests have not been ordered.

Approximately one week after finding out about fructose, I called my local specialist and inquired about being given a hydrogen breath test.

I explained that this test and a couple of others were what the Augusta specialist had scheduled for me, but the response I received was less than stellar.

I was told they would not run the tests because they were considered nuclear medicine and were very expensive, which left me depressed but more determined to educate myself.

I recently read that a doctor who specialized in gastroenterology moved to New York City, he found that due to his emersion into a "Western" diet he experienced drastic reactions in his life. Soon after, he started to have symptoms of irritable bowel syndrome and depression. Becoming a patient of the system in which he was practicing was such a shock to him that it prompted him to search for an alternative solution to his health problems.

Many patients who have been told by their doctors that their conditions would require surgery and/or medication for the rest of their lives are now able to avoid the knife and to get rid of their medications completely.

I am not telling you to purchase a cleansing product or a detoxification treatment. I am telling you that by changing your eating habits, you can accomplish this on your own.

Within the first couple of weeks after I began changing my diet by following my Fructose-Specific Food Charts, my health started to improve rapidly. My fatigue, hunger, and pain started to disappear. My IBS was starting to vanish. My depression and brain fog lifted. My body seemed to reset itself. All of the irritation, moodiness, and low energy levels, allergies, and poor digestive function that I had been experiencing were connected to my gut.

As I continued to rip out fructose in my body I experienced a very clear mind, I could pay attention and stay focused, I felt full of energy; my skin cleared, my color was better. I felt better and younger than I had in years.

All of these things were different ways my body was trying to tell me that it was out of balance and toxic.

This was the missing part of my health puzzle, the untapped source of my healing identifying fructose in food and eradicating it from my diet.

The amount of fructose in prepared foods has grown to be a problem since the end of 1960. Primarily due to the invention and use of high fructose corn syrup (HFCS), fructose now threatens our physical and mental well-being.

Our bodies must re-train our brains as to "not forget" the value of our digestive tract.

Medical professionals have developed tunnel vision and have a fascination with molecules and microtechnology. They have targeted their attention obsessively on smaller and smaller aspects of our biology while losing interest in looking at the big picture, and that is getting to the root cause of your illness.

Not only did I reverse 95 % of my diseased condition, I also lost 50 pounds, found a new level of energy, and I felt good about each morning.

# My body began to heal itself!

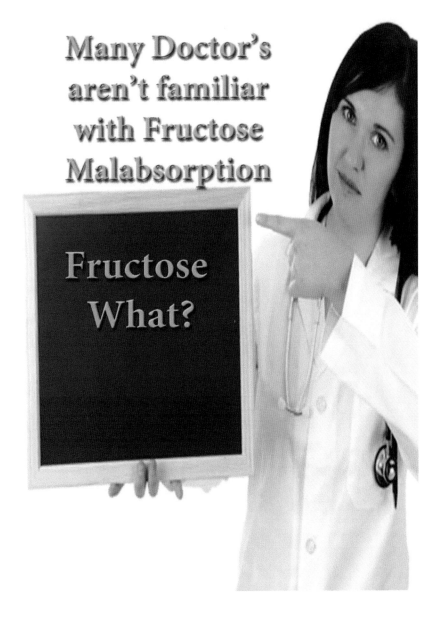

**Many Doctor's aren't familiar with Fructose Malabsorption**

**Fructose What?**

In Chapter 6, I will provide you with a concise picture of fructose, and High Fructose Corn Syrup and a means to improve your digestive health. You will learn how to identify, eradicate, and deal with your *fructose malabsorption* in a simple and effective way.

I have *Hereditary Fructose Intolerance* but *thousands* have *fructose malabsorption*!

Quick note:  Hereditary Fructose Intolerance- vs. – Fructose Malabsorption

For those individuals who think that when you state that Fructose Malabsorption and Hereditary Fructose Intolerance have the same issues…and they argue with you…they are only sharing with you the limited knowledge they have on the health issue.

1. Yes they are two separate health issues in this way…obviously one is hereditary which donates it is genetic and has more serious consequences. Mutations in the ALDOB gene cause HFI.
2. Yes they have the same symptoms
3. Yes they react to the same food selections
4. Yes either or will make you ill but only one will kill you
5. Yes testing is the same to determine either

For me to regain my health, I needed to be able to identify the *fructose* in my diet. That would be easier said than done.

 Advertising and the food conglomerates make sure it is not an easy task…it takes time to educate yourself so you know what you are and are not eating.  I soon found out that the problem wasn't just the fructose I digested from natural sources - the big problem was high fructose corn syrup (HFCS)!  HFCS is the moneymaker and the root of health problems for millions of people.  I needed to identify fructose and HFCS in my food.

I soon found out that what you see is not necessarily, what you get! Read the labels so you know what is in the product. It can literally save your life!

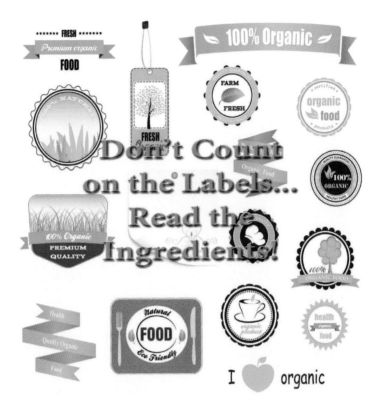

My Education Process!

My education continues but at the start of this book, I had over 3,000 pages of research.

From my initial discovery of finding out I had Hereditary Fructose Intolerance ...I wanted to know what was the clear concise way to eat so I could improve my health and all someone could give me was one piece of paper that was supposed to be something I could live by? Nope, that wasn't the answer.

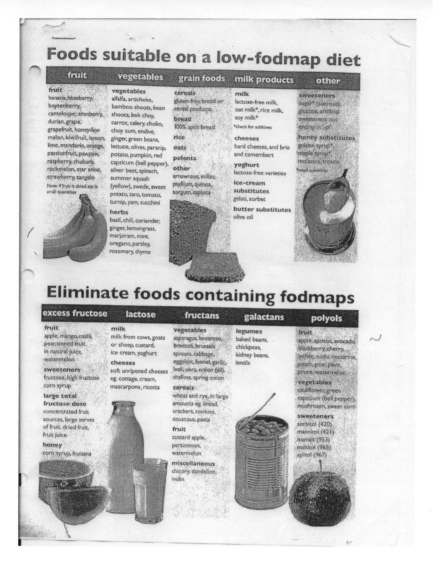

# Foods suitable on a low-fodmap diet

| fruit | vegetables | grain foods | milk products | other |
|---|---|---|---|---|
| **fruit**<br>banana, blueberry, boysenberry, cantaloupe, cranberry, durian, grape, grapefruit, honeydew melon, kiwifruit, lemon, lime, mandarin, orange, passionfruit, pawpaw, raspberry, rhubarb, rockmelon, star anise, strawberry, tangelo<br>Note: if fruit is dried, eat in small quantities | **vegetables**<br>alfalfa, artichoke, bamboo shoots, bean shoots, bok choy, carrot, celery, choko, choy sum, endive, ginger, green beans, lettuce, olives, parsnip, potato, pumpkin, red capsicum (bell pepper), silver beet, spinach, summer squash (yellow), swede, sweet potato, taro, tomato, turnip, yam, zucchini<br>**herbs**<br>basil, chili, coriander, ginger, lemongrass, marjoram, mint, oregano, parsley, rosemary, thyme | **cereals**<br>gluten-free bread or cereal products<br>**bread**<br>100% spelt bread<br>**rice**<br>**oats**<br>**polenta**<br>**other**<br>arrowroot, millet, psyllium, quinoa, sorghum, tapioca | **milk**<br>lactose-free milk, oat milk*, rice milk, soy milk*<br>*check for additives<br>**cheeses**<br>hard cheeses, and brie and camembert<br>**yoghurt**<br>lactose-free varieties<br>**ice-cream substitutes**<br>gelati, sorbet<br>**butter substitutes**<br>olive oil | **sweeteners**<br>sugar* (sucrose), glucose, artificial sweeteners not ending in '-ol'<br>**honey substitutes**<br>golden syrup*, maple syrup*, molasses, treacle<br>*small quantities |

# Eliminate foods containing fodmaps

| excess fructose | lactose | fructans | galactans | polyols |
|---|---|---|---|---|
| **fruit**<br>apple, mango, nashi, pear, tinned fruit in natural juice, watermelon<br>**sweeteners**<br>fructose, high fructose corn syrup<br>**large total fructose dose**<br>concentrated fruit sources, large serves of fruit, dried fruit, fruit juice<br>**honey**<br>corn syrup, fruisana | **milk**<br>milk from cows, goats or sheep, custard, ice cream, yoghurt<br>**cheeses**<br>soft unripened cheeses eg. cottage, cream, mascarpone, ricotta | **vegetables**<br>asparagus, beetroot, broccoli, brussels sprouts, cabbage, eggplant, fennel, garlic, leek, okra, onion (all), shallots, spring onion<br>**cereals**<br>wheat and rye, in large amounts eg. bread, crackers, cookies, couscous, pasta<br>**fruit**<br>custard apple, persimmon, watermelon<br>**miscellaneous**<br>chicory, dandelion, inulin | **legumes**<br>baked beans, chickpeas, kidney beans, lentils | **fruit**<br>apple, apricot, avocado, blackberry, cherry, lychee, nashi, nectarine, peach, pear, plum, prune, watermelon<br>**vegetables**<br>cauliflower, green capsicum (bell pepper), mushroom, sweet corn<br>**sweeteners**<br>sorbitol (420), mannitol (421), isomalt (953), maltitol (965), xylitol (967) |

The information in the above single piece of paper was all I had to go on and that was not comforting!

Therefore, the FODMAP was my catalyst for my research and was the beginning of how my food selections where decided.

FODMAP Definition: The term is an acronym, deriving from Fermentable, Oligo, Di, Mon-saccharides and Polyols. The restriction of the items listed on this page has been found to have a beneficial effect to sufferers or gastrointestinal disorders.

Why is it so damn confusing to the medical profession to figure out what food does or does not have fructose as a component of the food source?

Frankly, the FODMAP... wasn't acceptable. It did not provide enough information for me to live by. That is when the research went into overdrive. I found out who was the leader in the Fructose issue and narrowed it down to seven substantiated solid resources.

I went back to my doctor and asked him did he have a list that covered the seven lists I had found. He said there wasn't one. Therefore, that was the start of many late nights.

It was imperative for me to figure out what I needed to do regarding my diet and how could I achieve a well-researched list that could be supported by major medical research centers. How do you know my research is correct? My life depended on my results so only the top research centers in the country were a basis for my research.

The process was time consuming to say the least. In order to have a concise guide I took the time to develop a relationship with the sources to come up with a list I could live by. I created a spreadsheet with information from seven top University and/or research hospitals. This is where the mass confusion comes into play. There are approximately seven different "FODMAP's" and many of them don't agree with each other. Some tell you a food is ok...others tell you don't eat it. One will tell you a food selection can be decided on based on the portion size. That does not work for me.

My spreadsheet lists a food it is followed by whether it is tolerated or not tolerated and followed up by who approved or disapproved the food. I show you each research centers and/or university and whether they agree or disagree that, a specific food is suitable to eat.

You now have a list and the list provides the back up on where the information came from.

If six or seven out of the seven research centers agreed on the fact that it was permissible and would not create an issue if I digested it…it was then added to a tolerated column and if they collectively agreed that it was not a food you should eat it was placed in a not tolerated column.   You can see who agreed and who did not.

If a food seemed to split 50/50 I removed it from my initial list to prevent confusion.

If it was not on my approved list…I didn't eat it.  I was creating this as a tool for my health…I wasn't creating a product.  If it was OK to eat fine, however if it was on my don't eat list…the portion didn't matter I don't eat it.

You have so much "MIS-INFORMATION" that people are eating things that they shouldn't be eating based on the fact the source came from a company trying to sell a product.

I took my list further by running the food items through a National/International base that would list what each food was comprised of i.e. fiber, carbs, protein, fat and so on

Now I could tell how much fructose a food item did or did not have and the information was now producing a percentage of how much fructose was in natural foods.  My charts were looked over by GI specialists and they were found to be sound.  I could calculate my fructose consumption close to the grams.

Ninety days after I started eating what was specifically approved for a person with Hereditary Fructose Intolerance…I regained my life.  I no longer had to guess or wonder… I now had the tool to guide and maintain my health.

I named my list Fructose-Specific Foods because it was my bible when it came to eating properly. My definition of Fructose-Specific Foods: Foods approved to eat for anyone who is diagnosed with Hereditary Fructose Intolerance or Fructose Malabsorption.

I will not tell you that this is the only list in the world…it is not…it is the first list that provided me with a fair and unbiased comparison using information from Harvard Medical, Boston University, University of Iowa, Cleveland Clinic, Mayo Clinic, Oxford, 4 different FODMAP's and the American Society for Clinical Nutrition.

I will break down what HFCS is, where it comes from, and how long it has been used in our processed foods. You need to know what health issues have increased in conjunction with the consumption of HFCS.

Ingesting toxic chemicals and medications, especially antibiotics (medicine designed to kill bad bacteria, but which also wipe out the good bacteria over time) has altered the delicate balance in our guts in almost everyone.

This chapter will provide you with a thorough education about HFCS.

## Let's Start at the Beginning…What Is Fructose?

Fructose is a simple sugar found in fruits, berries and some vegetables; it has the same chemical formula as glucose, the simple sugar preferred by brain neurons.

That is, a molecule of either sugar contains six carbon atoms, six oxygen atoms and twelve hydrogen atoms. The difference between fructose and glucose lies in the arrangement of the atoms.

Glucose is dismantled very effectively by metabolic machinery of cells and produces abundant energy in a form cells can easily use. (13)

Fructose is also metabolized, but it follows a different pathway than glucose does (because of its different shape) and becomes a free fatty acid instead of being converted easily to energy for the cell.

Fructose is found in vegetables and fruits, which are natural and organically grown, but the fructose you get from food naturally is broken down in the body for the most part.

Your body can, and does, deal effectively with fructose, but only up to a point! The amount that can be effectively metabolized seems to be about 15-18 g of fructose per day.

### Definition of Fructose Malabsorption:

Fructose malabsorption, formerly named "dietary fructose intolerance," is a digestive disorder, unlike Hereditary Fructose Intolerance, which is a genetic health issue, in which absorption of fructose is impaired by deficient fructose carriers in the small intestines (entrecotes). This results in an increased concentration of fructose in the entire intestine.

### Why should you care about Fructose Malabsorption or HFCS in Your Food?

Fructose malabsorption affects over 100 million Americans, and most of them are led to believe they have Irritable Bowel Syndrome – a misdiagnosis that diminishes the quality of their life.

Thousands of people, particularly from western cultures, are currently suffering from many different digestive issues that are being lumped together as Irritable Bowel Syndrome.

### Isn't Fructose Natural?

Of course, it is…when it comes in the form of fruits and vegetables. So is sugar, so is vitamin D. So is alcohol. Being natural doesn't mean something is good for you. (14)

There are no rules about what may be labeled *natural*. *Natural* is just a word the food industry uses to make you feel good about the processed foods you eat.

Why we love the word *natural* is beyond me. Spider venom is natural; hurricanes, tsunamis, and tornadoes are natural. All the poisonous plants in the world are natural.

So when something is labeled *All Natural*, look a little closer at the label.

Sometimes the product will actually be a healthy choice, but most of the time not so much!

Read the fine print...your definition of *natural* may not match that of the product you are buying. As they say, "BUYER BEWARE"!

## What is High Fructose Corn Syrup?

High-fructose corn syrup (HFCS)—also called glucose/fructose in Canada, Isoglucose or Glucose-Fructose syrup and high-fructose maize syrup in other countries—comprises any of a group of corn syrups that has undergone enzymatic processing to convert some of its glucose into fructose to produce a desired sweetness. (14)

Due to US-imposed tariffs, in the United States sugar prices are two to three times higher than in the rest of the world, which makes HFCS significantly cheaper, so that it is the principal sweetener used in processed foods and beverages.

It is commonly used in breads, cereals, breakfast bars, lunch meats, yogurts, soft drinks, soups, and condiments.

HFCS consists of 24% water and the rest sugars.

## How is HFCS Produced?

HFCS was first introduced by Richard O. Marshall and Earl R. Kooi in 1957.

They were, however, unsuccessful in making it viable for mass production, primarily because the glucose-isomerizing activity they discovered required arsenite, which was highly toxic to humans.

The glucose (xylose) isomerase that did not require arsenite ion for its catalytic activity and thus was industrially feasible was first discovered by Dr. Key Yamanaka, Kagawa University, Japan, in 1961

HFCS is produced by milling corn (maize) to produce cornstarch, then processing that starch to yield corn syrup, which is almost entirely glucose, and then adding enzymes that change some of the glucose into fructose. The resulting syrup (after enzyme conversion) contains approximately 42% fructose and is HFCS 42. Some of the 42% fructose is then purified to 90% fructose, HFCS 90. To make HFCS 55, the HFCS 90 is mixed with HFCS 42 in the appropriate ratios to form the desired HFCS 55. (15)

## Why & When Was High Fructose Corn Syrup (HFCS) Introduced to Our Food?

Sucrose from sugar cane or sugar beets has been a part of the human diet for centuries; sucrose from fruit or honey has been a part of the human diet for millennia. Sucrose continues to be the benchmark against which other sweeteners are measured.

Notation: Sugar Beets were digested by the system when the entire beet was digested, it was tolerated because the beet had a great deal of fiber which helped the digestive system break this down...once man extracted the sugar from it...the fibrous part was discarded and provided sugar. Because of this process, the sugar from sugar beets is very hard to digest and provides issues with the Liver.

However, sucrose has posed significant technological problems in certain applications: it hydrolyzes in acidic systems, changing the sweetness and flavor characteristics of the product, and it is a granular ingredient that must be dissolved in water before use in many applications. (12)

Furthermore, sugar cane was traditionally grown in equatorial regions, some known equally well for both political and climatic instability.

The availability and price of sugar fluctuated wildly in response to upsets in either one.

Due to that increase in the price of sugar, many large companies compensated their costs in an effort to improve their bottom line by using "High Fructose Corn Syrup" to sweeten items such as but not limited to our soft drinks. It is currently used in thousands of products

It was toward the end of the 1960's that High Fructose Corn Syrup was rolled out to the public by food conglomerates.

HFCS immediately proved itself an attractive alternative to sucrose in liquid applications because it is stable in acidic foods and beverages.

Because it is syrup, HFCS can be pumped from delivery vehicles to storage and mixing tanks, requiring only simple dilution before use. As an ingredient derived from corn—a dependable, renewable, and abundant agricultural raw material of the US Midwest—HFCS has remained immune from the price and availability extremes of sucrose...it was principally for these reasons that HFCS was so readily accepted by the food industry and enjoyed such spectacular growth.

Because it is syrup, HFCS can be pumped from delivery vehicles to storage and mixing tanks, requiring only simple dilution before use.

## Does HFCS Come in Different Strengths?

Yes, HFCS exists in different grades, denoted by the percentage of fructose.

The Clinical Research Associate (CRA) claims that the grade used are HFCS-42 (42% fructose), and HFCS-55 which is used by the large "Cola" companies.

However, last year researchers assayed locally obtained bottled soda and found that three national brands had 65% fructose.

It gets worse. Cornsweet 90, a product of ADM, is HFCS-90. This intensely sweet HFCS is used for low-cal, low-fat products.

Why? The same sweetness can be imparted with fewer calories.

Sounds like a diet bargain until you realize that you're getting the bonus of extra fructose that can lead to liver problems, IBS, Type II Diabetes and other ailments, including obesity.

To close, crystalline fructose, now used in beverages like "Vitamin Water," is not fructose extracted from fruits and vegetables - it is a crystallized high grade HFCS. This HFCS has the upper limits of 90 to 95% fructose.

Fructose: whether it is called High Fructose Corn Syrup or given another name by our food industry, this substance has been increasingly used in canned, frozen, or prepared processed foods so much that we are poisoning ourselves and don't realize it. You can bet that if a product reads "New Improved Flavor" you are ingesting a great deal of fructose. (14)

Everyone needs to be educated about this "crap" we are unknowingly placing in our bodies and in the bodies of our children.

What Synonyms Does The Sugar Industry Use For HFCS When Labeling?

According to biochemist Russ Bianchi, HFCS is "intentionally mislabeled, or (uses) deceptively legally noncompliant names" that include chicory, inulin, iso-glucose, glucose-fructose syrup, dahlia syrup, tapioca syrup, glucose syrup, corn syrup, crystalline fructose, Inulin and (flat-out fraudulently) fruit fructose, or agave.

The most widely used varieties of HFCS are HFCS 55 (mostly used in soft drinks - approximately 55% fructose and 42% glucose) and HFCS 42 (used in beverages, processed foods, cereals, and baked goods - approximately 42% fructose and 53% glucose). HFCS-90 (approximately 90% fructose and 10% glucose) is used in small quantities for specialty applications but primarily is used to blend with HFCS 42 to make HFCS 55.

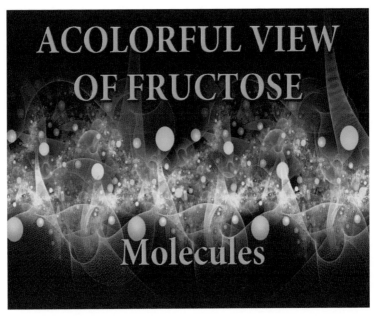

### I Have IBS...How Does That Relate to Fructose Malabsorption?

One doctor in Augusta, pioneer in researching the association between fructose malabsorption and IBS symptoms, has been hard at work educating his fellow GI specialists to test for and treat this ubiquitous problem; however, many doctors are not well versed on this emerging issue.

Since IBS causes non-specific symptoms of abdominal bloating, discomfort/pain, constipation, diarrhea, and gas, it is important for IBS problems to be fully evaluated - and this should include testing for poor digestion of dietary sugars like fructose, as well as for excess gut bacteria.

Four major research universities/centers support the fact that 65% of all Irritable Bowel Syndrome (IBS) patients actually suffer from fructose malabsorption. A simple test can support or rule out a diagnosis of fructose malabsorption.

Conversely, patients with fructose malabsorption often fit the profile of those with IBS. A small proportion of patients with both fructose malabsorption and lactose intolerance can suffer from celiac disease.

Fructose malabsorption is a condition in which the small intestine can't properly break down fabricated ADDITIVES (HFCS) so they are identified as a toxin by your liver and stored as fat. This is harmful to your liver, kidneys, and pancreas just for starters.

The doctor's team from Augusta has shown that of the patients who have come to their clinic at the University of Iowa Health Care suffering for IBS symptoms (gas, bloating, belching, nausea, indigestion, diarrhea, and abdominal discomfort/pain) over one third were found to have a fructose intolerance problem (malabsorption).

Further, they found there was a direct relationship between escalating digestive symptoms and increasing the test dose of fructose.

Symptoms of Fructose Malabsorption that Mirror HFI:

- Bloating (from fermentation in the small and large intestine)
- Diarrhea and/or constipation & Flatulence
- Stomach Pain (because of muscle spasms... the pain intensity of which can vary from mild and chronic to acute but erratic)
- Nausea
- Vomiting (if great quantities are consumed)
- Early signs of clinical mental depression
- Fuzzy head & Fatigue &Aching eyes
- Rapid weight gain or loss
- Symptoms of hypoglycemia: sugar craving, tremor, fainting, and in severe cases convulsions or coma

An enterocyte is a type of cell that absorbs water and nutrients from the digestive tract.

In the small intestine, they produce and secrete digestive enzymes, which bind to their brush borders and help break down sugars and proteins, making them small and easier to absorb. (16)

Enterocytes in the large intestine (colon) absorb water and electrolytes. In short, the ability to break down fructose is impaired so fructose molecules travel down to the large intestine without first being broken down; this situation can get ugly!

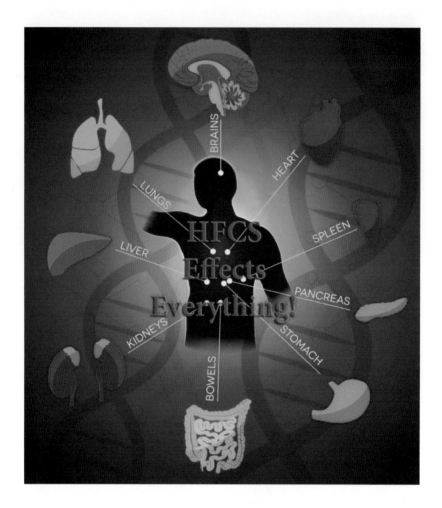

Which organs of the body are primarily affected by fructose/HFCS and how do these substances affect you as a sufferer of IBS.  Our digestive health plays a tremendous part in whether we are well nourished.

Our digestive tract is similar to the roots of a plant.  Both are not visible but both absorb water and nutrients, and when that "root" is sick both the root and the plant or in our case the intestines and the body demonstrate symptoms of organs far away from that root.

106

Fructose affects everything. As outlined in the diagram, it has a tremendous impact on many of our organs. Education regarding fructose/high fructose corn syrup is crucial to everyone. HFCS is a manufactured additive and the body can't break it down.

HFCS is a foreign substance and the liver processes this as fat. You need to know what can be affected and how it relates to you and/or your family! From your digestive tract to you memory...everything is affected by a fructose overload - it robs us of essential vitamins and minerals we need in order for our bodies to be healthy both mentally and physically.

## Is HFCS Harmful to Our Body?

Yes. High Fructose Corn Syrup is often singled out as Food Enemy No. 1 because it has become ubiquitous in processed foods over about the last 30 years...a period that coincides with a steep rise in obesity and many other illnesses that are discussed in this book.

Average American Consumption: The average American consumes approximately 120-160 grams of fructose a day. Our bodies were not made to digest this without severe consequences.

Considering that the average American drinks 50 gallons of soda and other sweetened beverages each year, it is important that we have more precise labeling on beverages. We need to be aware of how much HFCS we are digesting.

## Which Organs Are Affected First When Ingesting HFCS?

The digestive tract is the first place it hits! (17)

First, a quote from Dr. Kirby of the Cleveland Clinic: "We [gastroenterologists] agree that fructose malabsorption is something of a medical mystery. From an MD's standpoint, it's a very gray area."

He continues, "Fructose issues and Leaky Gut Syndrome is not a diagnosis taught in medical school … You hope that your doctor is a good-enough Sherlock Holmes, but sometimes it is very hard to make a diagnosis."

Dr Lee, another gastroenterologist from the Cleveland Clinic, states that, "We don't know a lot but we do know that it [fructose malabsorption] exists."

Both Dr. Lee and Dr. Kirby agree that gastroenterologists know that Hereditary Fructose Intolerance and fructose malabsorption exist, and that in-depth research is needed to provide help to those patients who have intolerance to fructose.

The human body has always known how to "detox" itself. It hasn't stopped and it hasn't changed…we have overloaded it with toxins.

Little is really known about your intestinal tract…and due to that lack of knowledge; many individuals will have to go through what I experienced.

Gastroenterologists are just beginning to understand many issues that plague their patients. Moreover, physicians don't know enough about the gut, which is the biggest immune system organ in the human body.

The path food takes through our guts follows the esophagus, the stomach, the small intestine (duodenum, then jejunum, then ileum), the large intestine (the colon and the rectum), and ends with the anus. Most of the digestive process occurs in the small intestine.

Fructose can only be metabolized by the liver and can't be used for energy by your body's cells.

It's therefore not only useless for the body, but is also a toxin and in high enough amounts, it creates a problem for the liver. The job of the liver is to get rid of it, and the liver mainly does that by transforming it into fat and sending that fat to our fat cells.

The body can break down some sugar naturally; however, this is not true for HFCS.

Fructose in any form (HFCS, sucrose, agave syrup) contributes to liver damage. Fructose is the most chemically reactive sugar.

Artificial sweeteners, especially in soft drinks, do not contribute dietary calories, but they apparently increase insulin production and contribute to hunger, eating, and obesity.

## HFCS Creates Chronic Inflammation which is a Corner Stone for Cancer

It creates chronic inflammation - a building block for Cancer.

Inflammation is the foundation for cancer and generative/autoimmune diseases. Small changes in diet and exercise (e.g. omega-3 oils, vitamin D, low starch, plant antioxidants, and maintaining muscle mass) can dramatically alter predisposition to disease and aging, and minimize the negative impact of genetic risks. Based on research regarding biological research, I am trying to explain how the anti-inflammatory diet and lifestyle combat disease.

Perhaps the better question would be what isn't impacted by an over-load of fructose or HFCS, Food Additives, Synthetic Inulin and GMO's

Our overall health issues can be affected by fructose or HFCS—it isn't just our gut!

Please note that the original information that continues to make its rounds on the internet was not from Johns Hopkins. I left this information in my book but added information so you realize that information must be weighed and measured against solid research.

This information was originally shared with me and it came from two sources…one…a doctor at Johns Hopkins and from a member of an on-line site that supports those with cancer. I found out the article did not come from Johns Hopkins but I left the article because you can go to valid research sites and find support for each of the bullet points.

Please read with an open mind and you decide what you need to take away from these points or what you just can't accept!

I have found solid support for several of the 15 of the items…we all need food for thought!

Note:  Number items in green are from the Internet Hoax from Johns Hopkins.  Items in blue are from solid research facilities and address the hoax.

1. Every person has cancer cells in the body. These cancer cells do not show up in the standard tests until they have multiplied to a few billion. When doctors tell cancer patients that there are no more cancer cells in their bodies after treatment, it just means the tests are unable to detect the cancer cells because they have not reached the detectable size.

**Does everyone have cancer cells in their body?**
**Everyone has cancer cells in their body, so why does one person never get cancer and other do?**

**There hundreds of reason why people develop cancer and there is not definitive answer as to point out only one source  however, a healthy immune system is a great defense when cancer happens.**

**Source:  Harvard Medical**

2. Cancer cells occur between 6 to more than 10 times in a person's lifetime.

I could find no solid support for this.

3 When the person's immune system is strong the cancer cells will be destroyed and prevented from multiplying and forming tumors.

This is what I could find from solid research centers on the connection of the immune system and Cancer.

What the Immune System Does

Your immune system is a collection of organs, special cells, and substances that help protect you from infections and some other diseases. Immune cells and the substances they make travel through your body to protect it from germs that cause infections. They also help protect you from cancer in some ways.

It may help to think of your body as a castle. Germs like viruses, bacteria, and parasites are like hostile, foreign armies that are not normally found in your body. They try to invade your body to use its resources, and they can hurt you in the process. Your immune system is your body's defense force. It helps keep invading germs out, or kills them if they do get into your body.

The immune system keeps track of all of the substances normally found in the body. Any new substance in the body that the immune system doesn't recognize raises an alarm, causing the immune system to attack it. Substances that cause an immune response are called *antigens*. The immune response can destroy anything containing the antigen, such as germs or cancer cells.

Germs have substances on their outer surfaces, such as certain proteins, that are not normally found in the human body. The immune system sees these foreign substances as antigens and attacks them.

Cancer cells are also different from normal cells in the body.

They sometimes have unusual substances on their outer surfaces that can act as antigens. However, germs are very different from normal human cells and are often easily seen as foreign, whereas cancer cells and normal cells have fewer clear differences. Because of this, the immune system doesn't always recognize cancer cells as foreign. Cancer cells are less like soldiers of an invading army and more like traitors within the ranks of the human cell population.

Clearly, there are limits on the immune system's ability to fight cancer on its own, because many people with healthy immune systems still develop cancer. Sometimes the immune system doesn't see the cancer cells as foreign because the cells are not different enough from normal cells. Sometimes the immune system recognizes the cancer cells, but the response might not be strong enough to destroy the cancer. Cancer cells themselves can also give off substances that keep the immune system in check.

To overcome this, researchers have found ways to help the immune system recognize cancer cells and strengthen its response so that it will destroy them.

Source: American Cancer Society.

TRAINING THE IMMUNE SYSTEM TO FIGHT CANCER

*July 2011*

Summary

Mayo researchers are exploring the hypothesis that the immune system plays a significant role in whether or not cancer cells proliferate. Their goal is to develop a cancer vaccine to boost the immune system.

The science crosses many disciplines and may develop new therapies for people with breast cancer, ovarian cancer and rheumatoid arthritis immunologist Keith Knutson, Ph.D., works across divisions in research to find answers.

The path from petri dish to prescription bottle is more like a bumpy dirt road than a superhighway. Because unearthing discoveries can require that researchers dig deep into one area of expertise, few ever see the entire stretch of road in their lifetime, leaving treacherous gaps between "basic science-land" and the mecca of the clinic. Enter Mayo Clinic immunologist <u>Keith L. Knutson, Ph.D.</u>, a rare breed of scientist who has made a career of bridging those gaps.

"Most of us are trained in one little corner of science, and it can be hard to look beyond that and reach out to researchers who are working in other domains," says Dr. Knutson's longtime collaborator <u>Sherine E. Gabriel, M.D.</u>"Keith has an appreciation and a respect for the entire breadth of research across the translational spectrum, and he looks for connections between his own work in the laboratory — which is world class — and patients in the clinic and people in the community. It seems to come naturally to him, though it is a challenge for many."

A running start

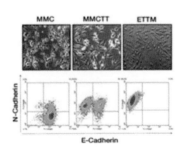

Dr. Knutson developed a culture method for generating pure populations of breast cancer stem cells using tumor necrosis factor-alpha (TNF-alpha) and transforming growth factor-beta (TGF-beta).

113

When combined, they cause transformation of breast cancer cells (MMC) into breast cancer stem cells (ETTM), which are stable in culture and can be studied. MMCTT cells are intermediaries between MMC and ETTM cells. His lab is developing vaccine strategies to target breast cancer stem cells.

One of the latest targets of this collaborative culture is cancer vaccines, which can train the body's own immune system to fight the disease. Many scientists believe that cancer cells arise and are destroyed by the immune system at an alarming rate, with cancer prevailing only when the immune system fails to do its job. This theory of basic biology is being applied to create a new generation of therapies that could revolutionize cancer care.

"We could use the same tactic that eradicated smallpox and other infectious diseases and apply it to cancer," says Dr. Knutson. "We may not totally eradicate cancer, but we hope that by boosting the immune system we could at least give the body a running start in preventing a tumor from growing unchecked." This disease approach is not new for him. Previously, at the University of Washington, his work led to vaccines that are currently being tested in clinical trials to prevent breast cancer relapse. At Mayo, his translational research has already led to two Mayo-industry collaborations aimed at moving two vaccines into people with breast cancer.

The immune system may already play an integral part of current cancer-fighting therapies. For example, the drug Herceptin targets a protein called HER2, which is more abundant on the surface of some breast cancer cells than on normal cells. What isn't clear is if, in addition to directly attacking the cancer cells, the drug also boosts the immune system to send more "soldiers" into the fight.

If the researchers find Herceptin works by bumping up the production of antibodies and that those changes are correlated with clinical outcomes, then the drug could be tweaked in the laboratory to make the treatment even more effective against cancer. That tactic is necessary because even though Derived stem cells can form tumor-like nodules in culture. These are useful to identify proteins and other molecules responsible for tumor growth.

Just as a boosted immune system could be more effective in fighting cancer, an impaired immune response could make people more susceptible to the disease. Researchers have shown that ovarian cancer "escapes" the body's defenses by actively suppressing the immune system, but no one has ever linked that laboratory finding with patients' actual responses to treatment. In addition, once women are diagnosed with ovarian cancer, there is wide variation in how people are affected, though it is not clear why.

*For the entire article, please see source*

Source: http://www.mayo.edu/research/discoverys-edge/training-immune-system-fight-cancer

How to Boost Your Immune System

What can you do?

Overall, your immune system does a remarkable job of defending you against disease-causing microorganisms. Nevertheless, sometimes it fails: A germ invades successfully and makes you sick. Is it possible to intervene in this process and make your immune system stronger? What if you improve your diet? Take certain vitamins or herbal preparations? Make other lifestyle changes in the hope of producing a near-perfect immune response?

The idea of boosting your immunity is enticing, but the ability to do so has proved elusive for several reasons. The immune system is precisely that — a system, not a single entity.

To function well, it requires balance and harmony.

There is still much that researchers don't know about the intricacies and interconnectedness of the immune response. For now, there are no scientifically proven direct links between lifestyle and enhanced immune function.

But that doesn't mean the effects of lifestyle on the immune system aren't intriguing and shouldn't be studied. Quite a number of researchers are exploring the effects of diet, exercise, age, psychological stress, herbal supplements, and other factors on the immune response, both in animals and in humans. Although interesting results are emerging, thus far they can only be considered preliminary. That's because researchers are still trying to understand how the immune system works and how to interpret measurements of immune function. The following sections summarize some of the most active areas of research into these topics. In the meantime, general healthy-living strategies are a good way to start giving your immune system the upper hand.

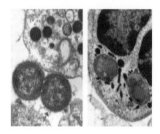

Immunity in action. A healthy immune system can defeat invading pathogens as shown above, where two bacteria that cause gonorrhea are no match for the large phagocyte, called a neutrophil that engulfs and kills them (see arrows). *Photos courtesy of Michael N. Starnbach, Ph.D., Harvard Medical School Source: Harvard Medical*

People who have problems with their immune systems are more likely to get some types of cancer. This group includes people who

- Have had organ transplants and take drugs to suppress their immune systems to stop organ rejection
- Have HIV or AIDS
- Are born with rare medical syndromes which affect their immunity

The types of cancers that affect these groups of people fall into 2 overlapping groups

- Cancers that are caused by viruses, such as cervical cancer and other cancers of the genital or anal area, some lymphomas, liver cancer and stomach cancer
- Lymphomas

Chronic infections or transplanted organs can continually stimulate cells to divide. This continual cell division means that immune cells are more likely to develop genetic faults and develop into lymphomas.

Source: http://www.cancerresearchuk.org/about-cancer/cancers-in-general/causes-symptoms/causes/what-causes-cancer

- When a person has cancer it indicates, the person has multiple nutritional deficiencies. These could be due to genetic, environmental, food and lifestyle factors.

- To overcome the multiple nutritional deficiencies, changing diet and including supplements will strengthen the immune system.

Both of these issues were answered in the Immune system section above.

6. Chemotherapy <u>involves poisoning</u> the rapidly-growing cancer cells and also destroys rapidly-growing healthy cells in the bone marrow, gastrointestinal tract etc, and can cause organ damage, like liver, kidneys, heart, lungs etc.

7. Radiation while destroying cancer cells <u>also</u> burns, scars and damages healthy cells, tissues and organs.

8. Initial treatment with chemotherapy and radiation will often reduce tumor size. However, prolonged use of chemotherapy and radiation do not result in more tumor destruction.

9. When the body has too much toxic burden from chemotherapy and radiation the immune system is either compromised or destroyed, hence the person can succumb to various kinds of infections and complications.

10. Chemotherapy and radiation can cause cancer cells to mutate and become resistant and difficult to destroy. Surgery <u>can also</u> cause cancer cells to spread to other sites.

**For 6-10 I would like to think is common sense. Of Course Chemotherapy is hard on the body but for many it is their only hope.**

Cancer cells cannot thrive in an oxygenated environment. <u>Exercising daily</u> and <u>deep breathing help</u> to get more oxygen down to the cellular level. Oxygen therapy is another means employed to destroy cancer cells.

Oxygen Therapy

**Other common name(s):** oxygenation therapy, hyper oxygenation, bio-oxidative therapy, oxidative therapy, ozone therapy, autohemotherapy, hydrogen peroxide therapy, oxidology, oxymedicine, germanium sesquioxide

**Scientific/medical name(s):** $O_3$ (ozone), $H_2O_2$ (hydrogen peroxide)

Description

Oxygen therapy introduces substances into the body that are supposed to release oxygen. The extra oxygen is believed to increase the body's ability to destroy disease-causing cells. Two of the most common compounds used in oxygen therapy are hydrogen peroxide and ozone—a chemically active form of oxygen. This type of treatment is different from the common medical uses of oxygen, which involve increasing the amount of oxygen gas in inhaled air. It is also different from hyperbaric oxygen, which involves the use of pressurized oxygen gas (see our document on _Hyperbaric Oxygen Therapy_).

Overview

Available scientific evidence does not support claims that putting oxygen-releasing chemicals into a person's body is effective in treating cancer. Some types of oxygen treatment may even be dangerous; there have been reports of serious illness and death from hydrogen peroxide. Ozone is a strong oxidant that can damage cells, and has also caused deaths.

Use of ozone or peroxide in small amounts under controlled conditions for treating limited parts of the body has shown some success in mainstream medical research studies.

How is it promoted for use?

Different varieties of <u>oxygen therapy are promoted as alternative</u> <u>treatments for dozens of diseases, including certain types of cancer,</u> asthma, emphysema, AIDS, arthritis, heart and vascular diseases, multiple sclerosis, and Alzheimer's disease.

Some supporters claim that cancer cells thrive in low-oxygen environments. They believe adding oxygen to the body creates an oxygen-rich condition in which cancer cells cannot survive.

Supporters of this type of treatment claim that it increases the efficiency of all cells in the body and increases energy, promotes the production of antioxidants, and enhances the immune system. A few proponents believe that soaking an affected body part can cause tumors to separate from the body so that a cancer can be "wiped away."

Source
http://www.cancer.org/treatment/treatmentsandsideeffects/compleme ntaryandalternativemedicine/pharmacologicalandbiologicaltreatment/ oxygen-therapy?sitearea=ETO

## Type II Diabetes

This is a chronic disorder of metabolism due either to partial or total lack of insulin secretion by the pancreas or the inability of insulin to function normally in the body.

Type II diabetes is an adult onset of diabetes. Type II may be precipitated by obesity, severe stress, pregnancy and other factors.

Insulin production removes glucose from the blood, e.g. lowers blood sugar, by increasing glucose transport into the fat cells.

If glucose is in your blood, but insulin is not present, e.g. type I diabetes, then you get thin.

If glucose is in your blood and insulin is present, then you get fat. If you are fat, glucose is still high in the blood, and insulin is present, then the fat cells will die unless they shut off the insulin response, i.e. insulin resistance.

Lowering the amount of carbohydrates, sweeteners/starch, in your diet makes it easier to control blood sugar levels and avoid hunger.

Research has shown consumption of HFCS and the over consumption of other sugars to be a leading factor in health decline with an increase of Type II Diabetes being part of the decline.

HFCS is absorbed more rapidly than regular sugar, and doesn't stimulate insulin or leptin production, which prevents your body from triggering the signals for being full and will lead to overconsumption of total calories.

Carbohydrates are not needed in your diet, since your liver can make all the blood sugar that you need from fats and protein. Most diabetics can benefit from a low carbohydrate diet.

Glucose, the blood sugar, is primarily responsible for turning on insulin production, so sweeteners (glucose, sucrose, HFCS, corn syrup) or dietary carbohydrates (starch, e.g. cereal, rice, pasta, potatoes, and bananas) that are readily converted to glucose can cause blood insulin levels to rise.

## Insulin Resistance

As fat cells accumulate, glucose because of blood sugar transported into the cells in response to insulin, more and more of the glucose is converted into fructose and on to pyruvate.

The pyruvate accumulates in mitochondria and ATP production is saturated.

This is potentially lethal for the cells, because the conversion of pyruvate into ATP is accomplished by removing high-energy electrons as the pyruvate is converted to carbon dioxide.

The high-energy electrons accumulate in the inner membranes of the mitochondria and if they are not systematically converted to low energy electrons and dumped onto oxygen to produce water, reactive oxygen species,

ROS are produced and the result is inflammatory oxidative stress. Antioxidants would be needed to protect from major cellular and organ damage.

The cells protect themselves by responding to the accumulation of high energy electrons on the mitochondria by shutting down the response to insulin and blocking further intracellular glucose accumulation. This is insulin resistance.

As you know, high blood sugar is bad for you but HFCS is so much worse!

One more thing to worry about...AGE stands for... Advanced Glycation End Products and it is tied to Fructose.

## What is Glycation?

High levels of blood sugar, glucose, react with proteins to produce advanced glycation end product AGE.

Fructose in the blood produces these inflammatory compounds more than ten times faster. That is why fructose is a bad sweetener for diabetics.

Corn syrup is not as sweet as pure glucose, because the syrup contains a mixture of short chains of glucose of different lengths, and the chains decrease in sweetness with length. By changing some of the glucose into fructose, the HFCS can be made as sweet as table sugar, sucrose.

Corn subsidies keep corn syrup cheap and make HFCS very profitable. Unfortunately, the HFCS contains fructose and therefore it has the liver toxicity and AGE-forming inflammation of fructose.

### How does AGE's affect our Aging?

*Do You Want to Have a More Youthful Appearance?*

*Fructose Will Age You in Many Ways!*

Cutting Costs is what big business is about and fructose costs less than other sweeteners. The food conglomerates have a budget and revenue will always trump your health!

*When you speak of Fructose and AGE, you are talking two different AGES'*

Fructose consumption will make you look older!

AGE—this age is the product of glycation reactions, in which a sugar molecule bonds to either a protein or a lipid molecule without an enzyme to control the reaction. Glycation is a haphazard process that impairs the functioning of biomolecules. (19)

### Aging

HAIFA, Israel, November 24, 1998 -- Researchers at the Technion-Israel Institute of Technology have shown in animal studies that excessive consumption of fructose, a sweetener, accelerates processes related to aging. Dr. Moshe Werman and Boaz Levi of the Faculty of Food Engineering and Biotechnology published their findings in the September 1998 Journal of Nutrition. (20)

## Fructose Increases the Rate of Aging—by William Misner, PhD

Dr. William Misner, PhD advises consumers to limit fructose intake to only natural fruits. No research associates whole fruit intake with health issues. There is general agreement that dietary fruit and vegetables are associated with optimal health. However, when live cells are exposed to processed form of fructose, the rate of aging increases dramatically. Skin is the largest organ it may profile the state of both external and internal health in man and beast. (21)

Werman & Boaz provide evidence that fructose and its phosphate metabolites can modify DNA faster than glucose and its phosphate metabolites under in vitro conditions.

These scientists report that cell structures of animals fed fructose aged more rapidly and accelerated aging of the collagen content of the skin also occurred.

Their data suggest that long-term fructose consumption induces adverse effects on aging; further studies are required.

## The Aging Process

The second major problem with fructose is its ability to combine with amino acids to form advanced glycation end products (AGEs). AGEs are believed to be permanent. They accumulate in body tissues where they accelerate aging and thus contribute to the formation of cataracts, narrowing of arteries and kidney disease.

Scientists have confirmed the damage to cells by the glycation process is irreversible. Fructose causes inflammation, which is implicated in most chronic diseases. Aging occurs from different mechanisms. However, the pathway to debilitating aging lies in our processed foods via High Fructose Corn Syrup! (22)

## How Fructose Accelerates Aging

Fructose adversely affects your body in a number of ways, but one of the mechanisms that cause significant damage is glycation, a process by which the sugar bonds with proteins and forms so-called advanced glycation end products, or AGEs. It's a fitting acronym because--along with oxidation--it's one of the major molecular mechanisms whereby damage accrues in your body, which leads to disease, aging and eventually death. (23)

### Liver

The human body handles glucose and fructose — the most abundant sugars in our diet — in different ways. Virtually every cell in the body can break down glucose for energy.

Eating fructose, e.g. agave syrup or sucrose, doesn't directly raise blood sugar/glucose levels, since it raises blood fructose levels, which is worse. Fructose is rapidly absorbed in the intestines and transported to the liver. The blood vessels of the liver remove fructose from the blood and it is then rapidly converted into fat. Fructose in sweeteners has now surpassed alcohol as the major source of liver disease.

Fructose is ten times sweeter than glucose, and that is why cheap forms of glucose, such as corn syrup, are treated with enzymes to convert some of their glucose into fructose to produce high fructose corn syrup.

About the only cells that can handle fructose are liver cells. What the liver does with fructose, especially when there is too much in the diet, has potentially dangerous consequences for the liver, the arteries, and the heart.

The entry of fructose into the liver kicks off a series of complex chemical transformations.

One remarkable change is that the liver uses fructose, a carbohydrate, to create fat.

This process is called lipogenesis. Give the liver enough fructose, and tiny fat droplets begin to accumulate in liver cells.

This buildup is called nonalcoholic fatty liver disease, because it looks just like what happens in the Livers of people who drink too much alcohol.

AGE...enzyme-controlled addition of sugars to protein or lipid molecules is termed glycosylation; glycation is a haphazard process that impairs the functioning of biomolecules, whereas glycosylation occurs at defined sites on the target molecule and is required in order for the molecule to function.

Much of the early laboratory research work on fructose glycations used inaccurate assay techniques that led to drastic underestimation of *the importance of fructose* in glycation.

Kidney/Fructose

A new study suggests that even individuals with normal kidney function are at risk for damage if they drink too much soda and soft drinks sweetened with high-fructose corn syrup may be the most dangerous.  Fructose is sweeter than glucose, and doesn't cause feelings of satiety, which may in turn cause damage via a different pathway than glucose. Instead of increasing blood-sugar levels, fructose may affect the kidneys

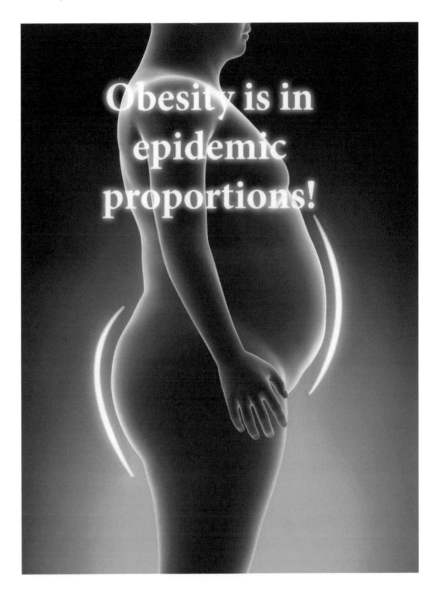

Researchers have long suspected that increased consumption of food flavored with fructose, a substance sweeter to the taste than glucose, may contribute to the U.S. obesity epidemic.

The brain requires glucose as a fuel. When there isn't enough in the body, it turns on cells to try to get a person to eat more. Once glucose levels rise, the brain turns those cells off.

Recent studies support the fact that fructose doesn't have the ability to operate that off switch.

Obesity is a worldwide 'epidemic'; when this term is used; it really is not used out of context or in a manner that is intended to create hysteria. All you have to do is to look around you and you can see what is happening. Let's face the reality: this 'epidemic' is as much about human nature as it is about the food companies using ingredients in the foods we eat to make them taste better.

During the last 30 years, obesity rates have more than tripled and diabetes incidence has increased more than seven fold. Perhaps this is not the only cause but a fact that cannot be ignored.

## Depression/Fructose

Researchers have found that those free floating fructose molecules actually react chemically with tryptophan, the precursor to serotonin, one of the neurotransmitters that help us feel happy, by degrading it and lowering serum levels.  (24)

## What is Tryptophan?

Tryptophan is one of the 10 essential amino acids that the body uses to synthesize the proteins it needs.

It's well known for its role in the production of nervous system messengers, especially those related to relaxation, restfulness, and sleep.  Remember…without tryptophan we feel depressed, irritable and angry.

For the sake of discussion, I'm going to condense depression, depleted zinc, and folic acid levels together.

Fructose/HFCS depletes key vitamins from our diet and doing so, it has a domino effect on our emotional well-being.

Depression may be more common in both adults and children with fructose malabsorption, and can improve with strict dietary reduction in fructose intake.

Fructose lowers the zinc, folic acid, and tryptophan levels in the blood, which cascade into multiple issues.

Zinc and folic acid blood concentrations have been reported to be decreased in a proportion of fructose intolerant individuals.

Ask your doctor to consider zinc deficiency when evaluating your symptoms suggestive of depression.

It is a surprisingly common but often overlooked factor that, when corrected through supplementation, can have profound positive effects.

Zinc is an essential component in modulating inflammation. A growing number of researchers and clinicians are beginning to recognize that there is a chronic inflammatory component in the etiology of depression.

So how did your brain cells forget their own chemistry? You need to find out how and why because that is the real diagnosis.

## The Serotonin Hypothesis

For the past 40 years, depressed mood has been thought to reflect lower levels of serotonin or lower sensitivity to it. Serotonin is synthesized from an amino acid precursor, tryptophan, which must be absorbed through digestion.

## Depression as Inflammation...As They Say in the Ads "DEPRESSION" Hurts!

A prominent alternate depression hypothesis postulates that the illness is actually the result of widespread inflammation throughout the body.

The process necessary for zinc assimilation may be the key to understanding and linking inflammation with this mineral deficiency.

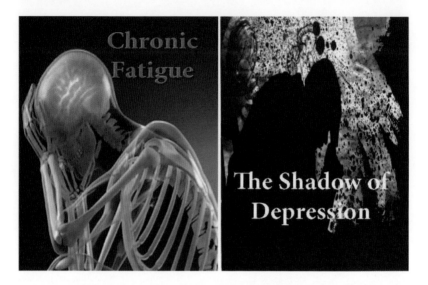

Zinc is one such mineral, and mounting experimental evidence indicates that it plays a central role in many metabolic processes relevant to the prevention and treatment of depression.

Folic Acid or B9

Vitamin B9, also called folate or folic acid, is one of 8 B vitamins. All B vitamins help the body convert food (carbohydrates) into fuel (glucose), which is used to produce energy. These B vitamins often referred to as B complex vitamins, also help the body use fats and protein.

B complex vitamins are needed for healthy skin, hair, eyes, and liver. They also help the nervous system function properly.

Folic acid is the synthetic form of B9, found in supplements and fortified foods, while folate occurs naturally in foods.

All the B vitamins are water-soluble, meaning that the body does not store them.

Folic acid is crucial for proper brain function and plays an important role in mental and emotional health. It aids in the production of DNA and RNA, the body's genetic material, and is especially important when cells and tissues are growing rapidly, such as in infancy, adolescence, and pregnancy.

Folic acid also works closely with vitamin B12 to help make red blood cells and help ironwork properly in the body.

Vitamin B9 works with vitamins B6, B12, and other nutrients to control blood levels of the amino acid homocysteine. High levels of homocysteine are associated with heart disease.

Alcoholism, inflammatory bowel disease, and celiac disease can cause folic acid deficiency. In addition, certain medications may lower levels of folic acid in the body.

The evidence about whether folic acid can help relieve depression is mixed.

Some studies show that 15 – 38% of people with depression have low folate levels in their bodies, and those with very low levels tend to be the most depressed.

One study found that people who did not get better when taking antidepressants had low levels of folic acid.

Dietary Sources for Folic Acid: Rich sources of folate include spinach, dark leafy greens, asparagus, turnip, beets, and mustard greens, Brussels sprouts, lima beans, soybeans, beef liver, brewer's yeast, root vegetables, whole grains, wheat germ, bulgur wheat, kidney beans, white beans, lima beans, mung beans, salmon, orange juice, avocado, and milk. In addition, all grain and cereal products in the U.S. are fortified with folic acid. Caution: individuals with fructose malabsorption can't digest many of these foods.

Fructose also raises your uric acid levels—it typically generates uric acid within minutes of ingestion, which in turn can wreak havoc on your blood pressure, insulin production, and kidney function. (25)

The link between fructose and uric acid is so strong that you can actually use your uric acid levels as a marker for fructose toxicity.

As you know, two-thirds of the US population is overweight, and most of these people likely have uric acid levels well above 5.5. Some may even be closer to 10 or above. Measuring your uric acid levels is a very practical way to determine just how strict you need to be when it comes to your fructose consumption

For example, if you're passionate about fruit and typically eat large amounts of it, but find out you have a uric acid level above 4.5 then you may want to consider lowering your fruit consumption until you've optimized your uric acid levels, to avoid harming your body.

## What Are AGEs?  Advanced Glycation End

AGEs are the products of glycation reactions, in which a sugar molecule bonds to either a protein or a lipid molecule without an enzyme to control the reaction. Glycation is a haphazard process that impairs the functioning of biomolecules (26)

Considering the dramatic increase in sugar consumption over the past several decades, and the subsequent increase in fructose consumption (recall that most sweeteners are approximately 50% fructose), is there any question why we're seeing rising rates of heart disease, arthritis, and other inflammatory "diseases of aging"?

### What Do AGEs Do In The Body?

The body is able to handle AGEs, though very slowly. The half-life of AGEs is about double that of the average cell life, meaning that damage can persist for quite some time, especially in long-lived cells like nerve and brain cells, eye and collagen proteins, and DNA.

Here's a run-down of a few effects of AGEs, and how they are implicated in many age-related chronic diseases such as: Type II Diabetes Mellitus, cardiovascular disease, Alzheimer's disease, cancer, peripheral neuropathy, and other sensory losses such as deafness and blindness.

Damage by glycation results in stiffening of the collagen in the blood vessel walls, leading to high blood pressure and the glycations also cause weakening of the collagen in the blood vessels walls, which may lead to micro- or macro-aneurisms; this may cause strokes if in the brain.

### How Do I Protect Myself?

You can keep yourself safe from a toxic load of these compounds by following the suggestions listed:

- Keep blood sugar low with fresh foods; this will reduce sugar supplies available for glycation.
- Eat vegetables and fruits raw, boiled, or steamed. When eating raw, there is no formation of these compounds because there is no cooking, while boiling and steaming introduce water to the cooking process.
- Avoid processed carbohydrates and browned foods. Food conglomerates take steps to increase caramelization and browning in their foods, directly increasing the levels of AGEs in the foods.

Cook meats low and slow – higher temperatures produce more AGEs than longer cooking times at lower temperatures. Rare and medium-rare meats will have fewer AGEs than fully cooked meats.

In the end, if you're not eating well-done meats often and are sticking to vegetables and fruits for your carbs, you're unlikely to be taking in dangerous level of AGEs. The body can deal with these substances so long as it isn't overloaded with them.

## Current Health Issues: Associated with HFCS

- Type II Diabetes
- Liver Problems and or Kidney Problems
- Obesity
- Depression
- Depletes our Chelated Zinc levels
- Depletes our Folic Acid levels

## HFCS creates metabolic disturbances that regulate:

- Appetite
- Weight gain
- Heart disease
- Cancer
- Dementia
- Depression
- Chronic Diseases, Extreme Fatigue
- Depletes our Zinc levels, Depletes our Folic Acid levels
- Depletes our main energy source "ATPS

Read the labels. If a product has HFCS or RHFC or corn syrup in general as an ingredient on the label (not the advertising on the label…the actual ingredient section of the label, you will not want purchase or consume that product.

It is time for all of us to demand an explanation as to why HFCS or RHFCS is used in any of our food products!

Please remember that an over abundance of sugar is still unhealthy…getting the food companies to switch to "real" sugar is only part of the battle…cutting down on ALL sugars is what is needed. Junk food will still be junk food and will make you fat and unhealthy!

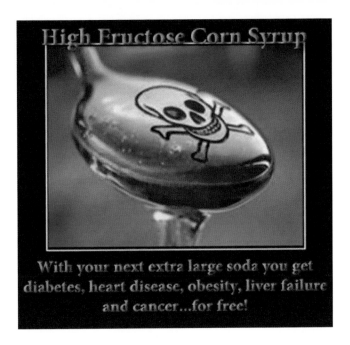

With your next extra large soda you get diabetes, heart disease, obesity, liver failure and cancer...for free!

Prior to Our HFCS Life:

In today's "fast-food lifestyle," we think our food and our schedules must compete with technology and the human body was never meant to compete with technology. We have carried over the attitude from our "High Tech" life that we must receive everything NOW.

We don't want to wait for anything so we grab what is quick even when we may be hurting ourselves. I was part of this process...I was as guilty as anyone was.

We, collectively, have helped create this monster due to our impatience and ignorance and it will take time and education on the part of both the patient and doctor to turn this health issue around in a positive direction.

I am in my 60's, so my Mother and my Grandmother cooked from scratch, and many of us had fresh food from home gardens, which to the most part do not exist today. I have retrieved many things from that life-style in order to reclaim my health.

I cook everything from scratch only using fresh or organic foods, which I purchase from Whole Foods, and no fructose comes into my home unless it is of an organic natural origin from fruits or vegetables that I can eat.

My point is…there is life after HFCS and it is so much better and to me and so much sweeter.

I previously mentioned that there is no magic bullet! Removing HFCS, RHFCS, or corn syrup in general is only part of the battle.

There is so much more to learn about fructose and the impact on our bodies.

I can assure you that I understand the pain, depression, and fatigue many of you face that has not been explained to you by your doctor.

We all have our own unique body chemistry, so there is not a "cure all" for everyone but I can promise you that by the time you finish my book you can have a healthier life and regain much if not all of your intestinal health and share the same success I have.

It is important for you to understand that the intestinal tract is in many ways one of the most important organs in the body. The majority underestimates the importance of intestinal health.

Other organs such as our heart, lungs, or brains seem to take center stage, and because both patients and doctors alike underestimate the intestinal tract, many of us can't seem to find the root of our health problems.

What happens when you can't find the cause? You are treated for your symptoms and your life will never be as robust as it was prior to your illness.

Treating your symptoms can only be temporary this can't be your long-term plan.

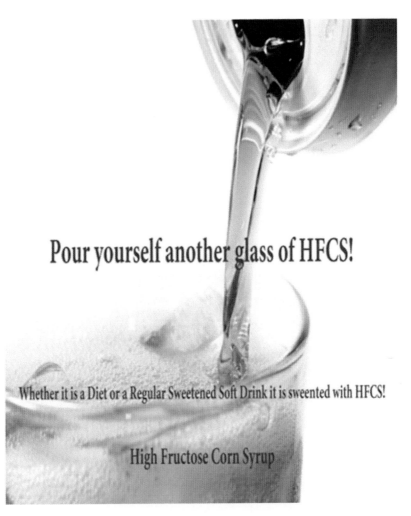

**Pour yourself another glass of HFCS!**

Whether it is a Diet or a Regular Sweetened Soft Drink it is sweented with HFCS!

High Fructose Corn Syrup

I found that the doctors and scientists of our country don't always agree but what I share with you in this chapter is accurate depiction of the HFCS problem currently facing our country. I know this because I lived and continue to live with this health issue. This information helped save my life. The following s a group of doctors and their scientific viewpoint in regards to HFCS. How the Corn Industry uses double talk to create confusion is purposely done. Food Conglomerates don't want to see anything happen to their "HFCS" because it will directly target their bottom line…PROFIT.

# IF YOU CAN'T CONVINCE THEM, CONFUSE THEM

– Harry Truman

Education on the subject of Fructose is vital because approximately 40% of our country is afflicted with a fructose malabsorption. When this substance was created…no one, knew the impact it would have 30 years later. I'm going to attempt to answer many of the possible questions and hope to clear the confusion on the difference of "Sugar" and High Fructose Corn Syrup (HFCS).

## What is the Current High Fructose Corn Syrup Debate About?

The current media debate about the benefits (or lack of harm) of high fructose corn syrup (HFCS) in our diet misses the obvious. The average American increased their consumption of HFCS (mostly from sugar sweetened drinks and processed food) from a couple of ounces to over 60 pounds per person per year.

Doubt and confusion are the currency of deception, and they sow the seeds of complacency.

These are used skillfully through massive print and television advertising campaigns by the Corn Refiners Association's attempt to dispel the "myth" that HFCS is harmful and assert through the opinion of "medical and nutrition experts" that it is no different from that of cane sugar.

HFCS is a "natural" product in the sense it is derived from corn .but it is manufactured. Except for one problem even when (HFCS) is used in moderation, it is a major cause of heart disease, obesity, cancer, dementia, liver failure, tooth decay and more.

## What reason does the Corn Industry have of misleading the public?

Why is the corn industry spending millions on misinformation campaigns to convince consumers and health care professionals of the safety of their product? Could it be that the food industry comprises 17 percent of our economy?

### The Lengths the Corn Industry Will Go To

The goal of the corn industry is to call into question any claim of harm from consuming high fructose corn syrup, and to confuse and deflect by calling their product natural "corn sugar." That's like calling tobacco in cigarettes natural herbal medicine.

### Medical Community & Corn Industry...What is the Connection?

Physicians are also targeted directly. I received a 12-page color glossy monograph from the Corn Refiners Association reviewing the "science" that HFCS was safe and no different than cane sugar.

I assume the other 700,000 physicians in America received the same propaganda at who knows what cost.

### Did the Corn Industry put a doctor on "Notice" for trying to educate the public?

Yes, some received a special "personal" letter from the Corn Refiners Association outlining every mention of the problems with HFCS in our diet – whether in print, blogs, books, radio, or television. They warned some doctors of the errors of their ways and put them on "notice."

## What Was the Response From These Doctors?

Their response was…what am I being put on notice for? I am not sure. To think they (Corn Industry) are tracking this (and me) that closely gives me an Orwellian chill.

## What Does the Corn Industry Do to Counter-Act This Vital Medical Information?

Any time information is posted or printed regarding the dangers of HFCS the Corn Industry conveniently creates or posts information directly around the warnings by creating new websites like www.sweetsurprise.com and www.cornsugar.com help "set us straight" about HFCS with quotes from professors of nutrition and medicine and thought leaders from Harvard and other stellar institutions.

Why is the corn industry spending millions on misinformation campaigns to convince consumers and health care professionals of the safety of their product? Could it be that the food industry comprises 17 percent of our economy?

### What Does Science Have to Say About HFCS?

What the Science Says about HFCS…Let's examine the science and insert some common sense into the conversation. These facts may indeed come as a sweet surprise.

The ads suggest getting your nutrition advice from your doctor (who, unfortunately, probably knows less about nutrition than most grandmothers do).

HFCS in promoting obesity, disease, and death across the globe that much has become clear.

Here are five reasons you should stay away from any product containing high fructose corn syrup. Moreover, in the opinion of a Harvard Doctor, it may kill you! (27)

1. Sugar in any form causes obesity and disease when consumed in pharmacologic doses. Cane sugar and high fructose corn syrup are indeed both harmful when consumed in pharmacologic doses of 140 pounds per person per year. `Species'

Our hunter-gatherer ancestors consumed the equivalent of 20 teaspoons per year, not per day. In this sense, I would agree with the corn industry that sugar is sugar. Quantity matters. Nevertheless, there are some important differences.

2. HFCS and cane sugar are NOT biochemically identical or processed the same way by the body. High fructose corn syrup is an industrial food product and far from "natural" or a naturally occurring substance. It is extracted from corn stalks through a process so secret that Archer Daniels Midland and Carghill would not allow the investigative journalist, Michael Pollan to observe it for his book, The Omnivore's Dilemma.

The sugars are extracted through a chemical enzymatic process resulting in a chemically and biologically novel compound called HFCS. Some basic biochemistry will help you understand this. Regular cane sugar (sucrose) is made of two-sugar molecules bound tightly together – glucose and fructose in equal amounts.

The enzymes in your digestive tract must break down the sucrose into glucose and fructose, which are then absorbed into the body.

HFCS also consists of glucose and fructose, not in a 50-50 ratio, but a 55-45 fructose to glucose ratio in an unbound form. Fructose is sweeter than glucose.

In addition, HFCS is cheaper than sugar because of the government farm bill corn subsidies. Products with HFCS are sweeter and cheaper than products made with cane sugar.

This allowed the average soda size to balloon from 8 ounces to 20 ounces with little financial costs to manufacturers but great human costs of increased obesity, diabetes, and chronic disease.

## Depletion of Our ATP:

This depletes the energy fuel source, or ATP, in our gut required to maintain the integrity of our intestinal lining. Little "tight junctions" cement each intestinal cell together preventing food and bacteria from "leaking" across the intestinal membrane and triggering an immune reaction and body wide inflammation.

ATP is the commonly used abbreviation for Adenosine Triphosphate. It is referred to as "nature's energizer." ATP is found in all cells and is the 'spark that lights the fire'.

In other words, it triggers cellular metabolism and with its presence, cells have no energy to repair, reproduce, or function.

In the case of skin cells, called 'fibroblasts', ATP is necessary for the fibroblasts to fulfill their role in producing collagen, the presence of which is characteristic of younger, healthier skin.

ATP also plays a secondary role in degrading and replacing damaged tissue whose presence often is the reason for signs of aging in the skin.

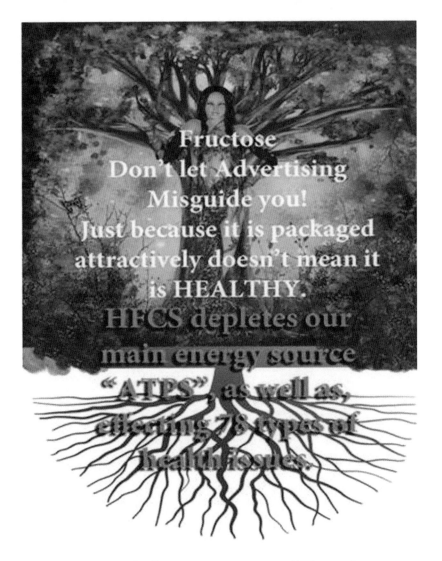

Fructose
Don't let Advertising
Misguide you!
Just because it is packaged
attractively doesn't mean it
is HEALTHY.
HFCS depletes our
main energy source
"ATPS", as well as,
effecting 78 types of
health issues.

For regeneration of cells or tissues to occur, ATP must be present, and the more abundant the presence of ATP, the greater is the potential for cells to repair and regenerate.

The result is a healthier, more productive, more youthful body, (or skin, in our case).

## Ladies...listen up...without ATP, you will look older!

High doses of free fructose have been proven trigger the inflammation that we know is at the root of accelerated aging.

3. HFCS contains contaminants including mercury that are not regulated or measured by the FDA. An FDA researcher asked corn producers to ship a barrel of high fructose corn syrup in order to test for contaminants. Her repeated requests were refused until she claimed she represented a newly created soft drink company.

She was then promptly shipped a big vat of HFCS that was used as part of the study that showed that HFCS often contains toxic levels of mercury because of chlor-alkali products used in its manufacturing.(i) Poisoned sugar is certainly not "natural".

When HFCS is run through a chemical analyzer or a chromatograph, strange chemical peaks show up that are not glucose or fructose. What are they? Who knows?

This certainly calls into question the purity of this processed form of super sugar.

The exact nature, effects, and toxicity of these funny compounds have not been fully explained, but shouldn't we be protected from the presence of untested chemical compounds in our food supply, especially when the contaminated food product comprises up to 15-20 percent of the average American's daily calorie intake?

- Independent medical and nutrition experts DO NOT support the
- Use of HFCS in our diet, despite the assertions of the corn industry.

Barry M. Popkin, Ph.D., Professor, Department of Nutrition, University of North Carolina at Chapel Hill, has published widely on the dangers of sugar-sweetened drinks and their contribution to the obesity epidemic.

In a review of HFCS in the American Journal of Clinical Nutrition, (ii) he explains the mechanism by which the free fructose may contribute to obesity.

It is further stated that, "The digestion, absorption, and metabolism of fructose differ from those of glucose. Hepatic metabolism of fructose favors de novo lipogenesis [production of fat in the liver].

In addition, unlike glucose, fructose does not stimulate insulin secretion or enhance leptin production.

Absorbed glucose and fructose differ in that glucose largely escapes first-pass removal by the liver, whereas fructose does not, resulting in different metabolic effects of these. These (HFCS) sugars serve as fertilizer for pathogenic bacteria, yeast and fungi, which crowd your good bacteria and upset the delicate balance of your gut. Discuss this issue along with Leptin-resistance the next time you see your Doctor. (28)

He states that HFCS is absorbed more rapidly than regular sugar, and that it doesn't stimulate insulin or leptin production.

The corn industry takes his comments out of context to support their position. "All sugar you eat is the same."

He was quoted as saying that "high fructose corn syrup is one of the most misunderstood products in the food industry."

When I asked him why he supported the corn industry, he told me he didn't and that his comments were taken totally out of context.

Misrepresenting science is one thing, misrepresenting scientists who have been at the forefront of the fight against obesity and high fructose sugar sweetened beverages is quite another.

5. HFCS is usually a marker of poor-quality, nutrient-poor disease creating industrial food products or "food-like substances." The last reason to avoid products that contain HFCS is that they are a marker for poor-quality, nutritionally depleted, processed industrial food full of empty calories and artificial ingredients. If you find "high fructose corn syrup" on the label, you can be sure it is not a whole, real, fresh food full of fiber, vitamins, minerals, phytonutrients, and antioxidants. Stay away if you want to stay healthy.

We still must reduce our overall consumption of sugar, but with this one simple dietary change, you can radically reduce your health risks and improve your health.

The real issues are only two.

- We are consuming HFCS and sugar in pharmacologic quantities never before experienced in human history — 140 pounds a year versus 20 teaspoons consumed more than a century ago.
- High fructose corn syrup is always found in very poor quality foods that are nutritionally vacuous and filled with all sorts of other disease promoting compounds, fats, salt, chemicals, and even mercury.

These critical ideas should be the heart of the national conversation, not the meaningless confusing ads and statements by the corn industry in the media and online that attempt to assure the public that the biochemistry of real sugar and industrially produced sugar from corn are the same.

Do you think there is an association between the introduction of HFCS in our diet and the obesity epidemic? What reason do you think the Corn Refiners Association has for running such ads and publishing websites like those listed in this article?

What do you think of the science presented here and the general effects of HFCS on the American diet?

To your good health… (29)

They say…what you don't know can't hurt you…unfortunately; many people are unaware of *Fructose Issues* and education could explain the struggle they go through each day with their digestive tract and how to improve their lives!

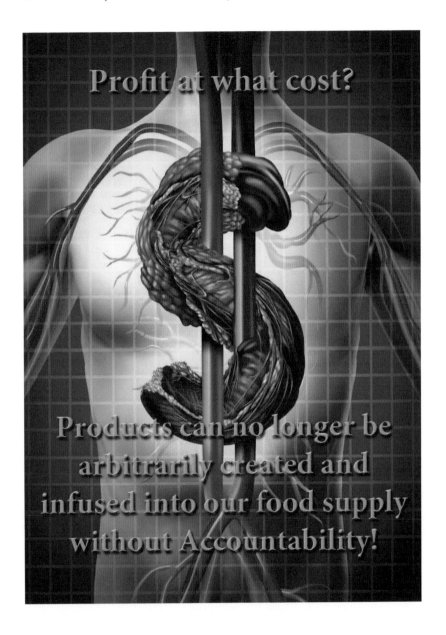

With this renewable and abundant way to increase, the bottom line there has to be some sort of accountability for the often-debilitating outcome of this product/ products!

As conglomerates are bringing in more and more money…HFCS and products like it are, being used more and more to bolster the bottom line with NO one being responsible,

How many people even looked at the possible long range affects of these fabricated additives?

As I look back at the 2 ½ years I lost…I realize that it was all due to benefit Corporate Profit…nothing else.  HFCS was created to decrease costs and improve profits.

How can the FDA stand back and not take a second look at High Fructose Corn Syrup, GMO's and other chemicals placed our food? What has to happen to get the FDA to revisit their original decisions?  Better yet, how did these items gain approval in the first place?

We depend on Department of <u>HEALTH</u> & <u>HUMAN</u> Services to provide us with safe and healthy items.  However, who is watching them?

Apparently, the status regarding the side effects from HFCS, GMO's, and Trans Fat doesn't seem to be bothering anyone at the FDA. What do they need for a wake-up call!

The Food and Agriculture Organization of the United Nations also says that farmers can grow more food on less land with genetically modified crops.

Genetically modified animals have certain genes inserted into their genomes so that they can produce 'better' milk, eggs, and meat.

The Genomes pass through the animals and products, end up in your digestive tract as indigestible properties, and create so many health issues.

I am hopeful people will take responsibility for their health issues by education.

## REMEMBER THE OLD ADAGE "WE ARE WHAT WE EAT"!

Well this statement is truer today than it ever has been in the past.

Our systems simply don't know how to process the chemicals so…we store this crap as fat and our "Fast Food, Quick and Ready to Eat products are creating more health hazards.

Our society doesn't seem to realize that when something is "Low Fat, Fat Free, or Sugar Free" that these items contain man-made/chemically engineered products and there is nothing healthy about placing these items in anyone's system. Thus the increase of Obesity, as well, as, an increase in the other serious health issues we are currently facing in our country.

Understanding the danger of fructose is not a passing phase. I have explained how HFCS affects our physical health…now I'm going to explain how it does and what influences both of our brains!

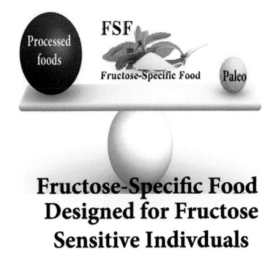

## Fructose-Specific Food Designed for Fructose Sensitive Indivduals

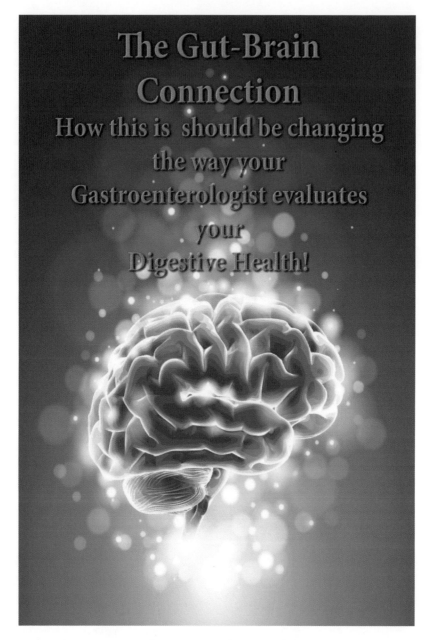

The Gut-Brain Connection
How this is should be changing the way your Gastroenterologist evaluates your Digestive Health!

Is this the missing link to many of our health issues? I support that theory that two major organs in our body are definitely linked!

Although I discussed this connection in previous chapters by briefly mentioning depression, the Gut Brain connection needs a chapter all on its own. This information makes sense and it supports the argument in regards to the connection of these two organs.

This information will explain many things that we feel physically as well as emotionally.

## The Brain-Gut Connection in IBS and Fructose Malabsorption.

Dysfunction in the connection between the brain and the gut may be a contributing factor in irritable bowel syndrome (IBS). Some health problems are simple to understand.

If you have a sore throat, your doctor will take a tissue sample from your throat and run a test to see if you have a strep infection.

A strange looking mole on your skin can be tested to see if it is cancerous. Unfortunately, IBS is far from simple. Unlike diseases that are visible, to understand what is going wrong in IBS, researchers have found that they need to look beyond the gut and toward the complex communication systems that connect the gut with the brain.

To appreciate the work that is being done in this area, I was told that you would need to have a degree in neuroscience. Well, I have no degree but I understand the information.

Even without such a degree, it is helpful to have some basic understanding of the complex connection between the brain and the gut, as well as, how this connection relates to IBS.

Have you ever had a "gut-wrenching" experience? Do certain situations make you "feel nauseous"? Have you ever felt "butterflies" in your stomach? We use these expressions for a reason.

The gastrointestinal tract is sensitive to emotion. Anger, anxiety, sadness, elation – all of these feeling (and others) can trigger symptoms in the gut.

The brain has a direct effect on the stomach. For example, the very thought of eating can release the stomach's juices before food gets there. This connection goes both ways.

A troubled intestine can send signals to the brain, just as a troubled brain can send signals to the gut.

Therefore, a person's stomach or intestinal distress can be the cause or the product of anxiety, stress, or depression. That's because the brain and the gastrointestinal (GI) system are intimately connected — so intimately that they should be viewed as one system.

This is especially true in cases where a person experiences gastrointestinal upset with no obvious physical cause. For such functional GI disorders, it is difficult to try to heal a distressed gut without considering the role of stress and emotion.

These factors – both emotional and physical needed to be identified before I could become healthy.

## Up the Down Staircase

Communication is a two-way street when it comes to the brain (central nervous system) and the digestive system (enteric nervous system). Complex pathways link the brain and the intestines with information flowing back and forth on a continual basis. This close connection is most clearly seen in our response to stress (perceived threat), which suggests that this complex communication network was very important for our survival as a species.

Nerves in the gut that are experiencing excessive sensitivity can trigger changes in the brain.

Thoughts, feelings, and activation of parts of the brain that have to do with anxiety or arousal, can stimulate exaggerated gut responses.

Malfunction may also be found along the many different pathways that connect the brain and gut.

For instance, there is evidence that abnormal functioning along two separate pathways in the autonomic nervous system is associated with the symptom of diarrhea vs. the symptom of constipation.

In general, it seems that dysfunction in the brain-gut communication system is interfering with the body's ability to maintain homeostasis, a state in which all systems are working smoothly.

The emerging and surprising view of how the enteric nervous system in our bellies goes far beyond just processing the food we eat. The second brain informs our state of mind in other more obscure ways, as well. As it is a big part of our emotions are probably influenced by the nerves in our gut.

The commonalities, like depression treatments can target the mind and unintentionally affect the gut. The enteric nervous system uses more than 30 neurotransmitters, just like the brain, and in fact, 95 percent of the body's serotonin is found in the bowels. (30)

## Stress and the Functional GI Disorders

Given how closely the gut and brain interact, it becomes easier to understand why you might feel nauseated before giving a presentation, or feel intestinal pain during times of stress.

Psychology combines with physical factors to cause pain and other bowel symptoms. Psychosocial factors influence the actual physiology of the gut, as well as symptoms.

In other words, stress (or depression or other psychological factors) can affect movement and contractions of the GI tract, cause inflammation, or make you more susceptible to infection.

Based on these observations, you might expect that at least some patients with functional GI conditions might improve with therapy to reduce stress or treat anxiety or depression.

# Is Stress Causing Your Symptoms?

Are your stomach problems, such as, heartburn, abdominal cramps, or loose stools …related to stress?

Watch for these other common symptoms of stress and discuss them with your doctor. Together you can come up with strategies to help you deal with the stressors in your life, and ease your digestive discomforts.

## Physical Symptoms:

- Stiff or tense muscles, especially in the neck and shoulders
- Headaches
- Sleep problems
- Shakiness or tremors
- Recent loss of interest in sex
- Weight loss or gain
- Restlessness

## Behavioral Symptoms

- Procrastination
- Grinding teeth
- Difficulty completing work assignments
- Changes in the amount of alcohol or food you consume
- Taking up smoking, or smoking more than usual
- Increased desire to be with or withdraw from others
- Rumination (frequent talking or brooding about stressful situations)

## Emotional Symptoms

- Crying
- Overwhelming sense of tension or pressure
- Trouble relaxing
- Nervousness
- Quick temper
- Depression
- Poor concentration
- Trouble remembering things
- Loss of sense of humor

Because antidepressant medications called selective serotonin reuptake inhibitors (SSRIs) increase serotonin levels, it's little wonder that meds meant to cause chemical changes in the mind often provoke GI issues as a side effect. Irritable bowel syndrome— that afflicts more than two million Americans—also increased in part from too much serotonin in our entrails, and this could be regarded as a "mental illness" of the second brain. (30)

## Different or Similar Symptoms, One Problem

### Autism and Fructose

Well over 10 to 15 years ago, you could have gone your entire life and never crossed paths with a child diagnosed with Autism and today it is nothing out of the ordinary! So, what has changed?

Scientists are learning that the serotonin made by the enteric nervous system might also play a role in more surprising diseases: In a new *Nature Medicine* study published online February 7, a drug that inhibited the release of serotonin from the gut counteracted the bone-deteriorating disease osteoporosis in postmenopausal rodents. (*Scientific American* is part of Nature Publishing Group.) (31)

It was totally unexpected that the gut would regulate bone mass to the extent that one could use this regulation to cure—at least in rodents—osteoporosis," says Gerard Karsenty, lead author of the study and chair of the Department of Genetics and Development at Columbia University Medical Center

So often, the effect of our contemporary diet makes itself known in a shocking way.

Toxins take the largest toll on children, their small body size means they've more affected by everyday amounts of toxin serotonin seeping from the second brain might even play some part in autism, the developmental disorder often first noticed in early childhood.

Gershon has discovered that the same genes involved in synapse formation between neurons in the brain are involved in the alimentary synapse formation.

If these genes are affected in autism," he says, "it could explain why so many kids with autism have GI motor abnormalities" in addition to elevated levels of gut-produced serotonin in their blood. (30)

Researchers explore how disruptions in the intestine's community of digestive bacteria may influence brain development and autism. (31)

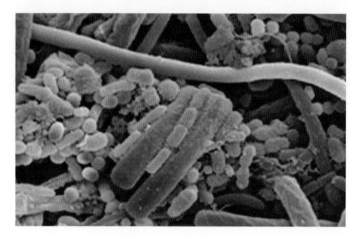

The intestinal tract is filled with billions of digestive bacteria essential for health. Autism researchers are exploring how disturbances in this community can affect brain development and/or worsen autism symptoms. (Colorized micrograph) (31)

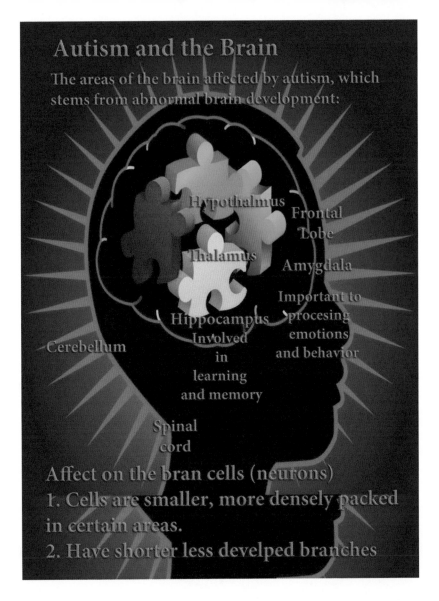

*How many parents want to take a risk with the health of their children?*

The idea of a gut-brain connection isn't new. It's supported by a large body of research showing continuous communication between the bacteria that inhabit the digestive tract and the body's immune system – and between the immune system and the brain.

A healthy gut microbiome exerts a calming effect on the immune system. In addition, some research suggests that byproducts from harmful gut bacteria can interfere with brain development and function. (31)

"We know clearly that many children with autism have GI problems, but we don't know exactly how those GI disturbances are related to brain function," comments Paul Wang, Autism Speaks vice president for medical research. "We need to understand the interplay between the gut and the brain so that we can identify the right treatment approaches." (31)

I would also include the rise in ADHD children…more now than 30 years ago!

## Alzheimer's Disease and Fructose

I read an article was of particular interest to me since my Mother died from Alzheimer's disease. You may not be convinced but it is something to ponder. The story certainly ties into my Fructose book. It provides additional information in health areas that I have not discussed. In addition, it provides another way to look at the Fructose problem.

A large body of evidence now suggests that Alzheimer's is primarily a metabolic disease. Some scientists have gone so far as to rename it: they call it type 3 diabetes.

New Scientist carried this story on its cover on 1 September.

Since then I've been trying to discover whether it stands up. I've now read dozens of papers on the subject, testing my cognitive powers to the limit as I've tried to get to grips with brain chemistry. Though the story is by no means complete, the evidence so far is compelling.

About 35 million people suffer from Alzheimer's disease worldwide; current projections, based on the rate at which the population ages, suggest that this will rise to 100 million by 2050. Nevertheless, if, as many scientists now believe, it is caused largely by the brain's impaired response to insulin, the numbers could rise much further. In the United States, the percentage of the population with type 2 diabetes, which is strongly linked to obesity, has almost trebled in 30 years. If Alzheimer's, or "type 3 diabetes", goes the same way, the potential for human suffering is incalculable.

In the United States, someone develops Alzheimer's disease every 69 seconds, and by 2050, this is expected to increase to a new case every 33 seconds, according to the Alzheimer's Association's 2011 Alzheimer's Disease Facts and Figures. (32)

Insulin is the hormone that prompts the liver, muscles and fat to absorb sugar from the blood. Type 2 diabetes is caused by excessive blood glucose, resulting either from a deficiency of insulin produced by the pancreas, or resistance to its signals by the organs that would usually take up the glucose.

The association between Alzheimer's and type 2 diabetes is long established: type 2 sufferers are two to three times more likely to be struck by this form of dementia than the general population. There are also associations between Alzheimer's and obesity and Alzheimer's and metabolic syndrome (a complex of diet-related pathologies).

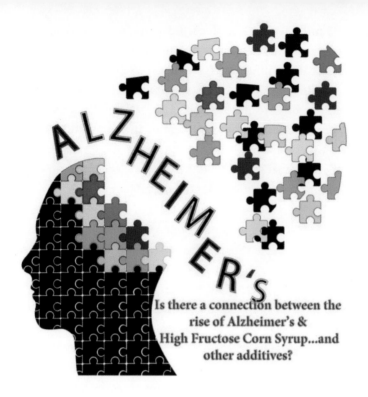

Is there a connection between the rise of Alzheimer's & High Fructose Corn Syrup...and other additives?

The disease is currently at epidemic proportions, with 5.4 million Americans—including one in eight people aged 65 and over—living with Alzheimer's disease. By 2050, this is expected to jump to 16 million, and in the next 20 years it is projected, that Alzheimer's will affect one in four Americans. If that happens, it would then be more prevalent than obesity and diabetes is today!

This certainly is a somber fact and if there is a direct correlation between Fructose and Alzheimer's research can't wait any longer to find out how far this additive can damage the human body!

- Vitamin D deficiency: In 2007 researchers at the University of Wisconsin uncovered strong links between low levels of vitamin D in Alzheimer's patients and poor outcomes on cognitive tests. Vitamin D may enhance the levels of important chemicals in your brain that protect your brain cells and combat the brain inflammation seen in dementia patients.

- Obesity, especially increased belly fat, insulin resistance, and diabetes: diabetics have up to 65 percent higher risk of developing Alzheimer's disease. Keep your fasting insulin level below three by minimizing sugar and grains and exercising regularly.

## Research is On Going or is it?

Fructose and fructans which are polymers of fructose are FODMAPs (Fermentable Oligo-, Di- and Mono-saccharides and Polyols) known to cause GI discomfort in susceptible individuals. A low FODMAP diet has widespread application for managing functional GI disorders such as IBS. This is likely the most education that any doctor currently provides to a patient like me...it may help a bit but so much more is needed. That is why there needs to be more dialogue and interest brought to the table so individuals can be educated about what they are eating and why it is slowly killing them.

## Fructose is the Next "Gluten Epidemic" on the Horizon!

You won't see the Gastroenterologist Centers in the country concentrate on this issue until you get... the American Gastroenterological Association behind the studies ...a direct quote from an associate who happens to be a gastroenterologist

I recently met with a Gastroenterologist to see if he may be able to take the time to write a forward for my book, he was kind and told me he would think about it.

However, as our conversation continued I wanted to know if there is a "Patient Advocacy" group in my area to educate people on Fructose Issues. He said very firmly, NO!

The doctor indicated that until the Gastroenterologist...American Gastroenterological Association (AGA) (as noted above) in general recognizes the Fructose Issue as collective group the issue of Fructose most likely will not be dealt with in a broad spectrum.

I inquired as to why and he said very honestly "There is no money in it" ...it being the education and study of diet changes due to Fructose.

I was shocked that after all my research and the personal connection and history I experienced with Fructose that no one was really pushing for educating the public.

I experienced first-hand how detrimental Fructose can be to your digestive system. How can our medical community not be more up to speed and why does our government seem to turn a blind eye toward this health issue? I thought that researchers would be pouring money into the impact of Fructose on the human body.

The public needs to know and we need to push for that education and awareness...if you educate someone and they refuse to learn or accept the information...you can rest that you have tried all that you could to help those individuals.

Currently many gastroenterologists don't recognize Fructose Malabsorption as an issue because there hasn't been enough research done for the specialists to stand united on this problem. Until that happens, you're not going to see a wide spread education program to assist patients with this health issue.

Every Gastroenterologist needs a nutritionist to work with their group and if this was the norm...the nutritionist would soon recognize what so many doctors don't want to look at and that is the "D" word...diet!

In the United States, Gastroenterology is an Internal Medicine Subspecialty certified by the American Board of Internal Medicine (ABIM) and the American Osteopathic Board of Internal Medicine (AOBIM).

Diseases affecting the gastrointestinal tract, which includes the organs from mouth to anus, along the alimentary canal, are the focus of this specialty.

A friend of mine told me that in her opinion the noble profession of "Doctor" has become more about the money and pharmaceuticals (for some) and less about finding the root of the illness.

She went on to state that "some" physicians are so closely tied to pharmaceutical companies that they are not going to suggest your problems may be coming from your acquired eating habits. That doctor's today aren't asking the "How" or "Why" they are more focused on technology and pharmaceuticals.

After all, if they fix you…they can't keep bringing you back for appointments and assisting the large pharmaceutical companies with added revenues.

She said, "Think about it…if all our doctors do is treat the symptoms we will never get better. If you never improve you continue your dependency on the Doctor—Drug cycle which, will continue forever."

I went from tri- monthly ER Visits and bi-monthly doctor visits (not counting the blood work or scans) to seeing a doctor once every 4 months and one prescription.

All of the changes that took place were due to diet. There is not a pill out on the market to fix what I was suffering from…diet was the only way to stop the nightmare.

Yet, no one every inquired about my diet or what I was eating.

*I recently had a chance to catch up with a very dear friend of mine… Yogi, he inquired how I was feeling and I told him I was much better…he stopped me from explaining any further…he simply asked me when was the last time I heard of a Doctor curing an illness…I paused for a moment and he said…I think it was Polio! He got me thinking about the question. He smiled and said that is why they call it a practice!*

# Medical care is tied to what you can afford!

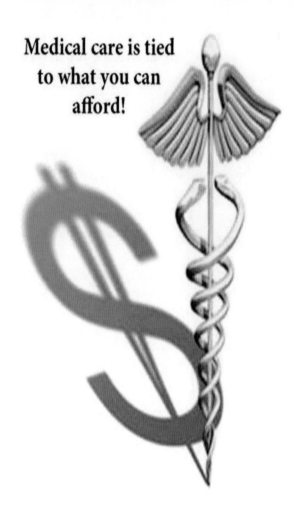

In all fairness to the medical community—Doctors are under the scrutiny and control of the Insurance companies and the government which in many instances ties their hands when they are trying to help diagnosis and treat their patients.

Our doctors are not permitted to practice as they have in the past due to the restrictions placed on them.

I respect the medical profession but each profession has its high achievers and—well—you must realize that includes those who aren't so good at what they do.

To prevent further inflammation and damage to our digestive tract we need to know how to prevent it.  We have been fed an overdose of chemically infused foods.  Education is key in order to find our way back to digestive health.  High Fructose Corn Syrup certainly tops our list but we have additional issues that compound your Fructose Malabsorption.  Inulin, Fructans, Prebiotics, Probiotics, and Sorbitol also play a role in how you feel and if these substances affect your "IBS" or other digestive disorders.

By understanding, the impact of these substances in conjunction with Fructose will provide you with a very thorough overview regarding how it ties into your digestive issues.

When I'm asked, "What can you eat?" My answer is not that simple. Obviously, proteins are not a problem, but how about fruits and vegetables and why can I digest say...shallots but not onions...aren't they the same?  Yes and No!  This question prompted me to include Fructans and Oligosaccharide intolerances in my book.

There is a reason why some fruits, vegetables, and grains can't be tolerated when you are dealing with a Fructose issue, whether it is from a hereditary standpoint or a malabsorption issue you need to add this to your information library.

## Inulin Another Food Additive:  Don't Confuse Inulin with Insulin!

What is Inulin? Inulin is a naturally occurring substance that helps keep the digestive system healthy. It can be found in foods such as bananas, onions, wheat and chicory root.

165

According to the National Cancer Institute, inulin helps healthy bacteria grow in the intestinal tract and helps with absorption of magnesium and calcium.

## Fiber

Inulin is non-digestible by human enzymes. It passes through the mouth, stomach, and small intestine without being metabolized. Because it is non-digestible, inulin is used as fiber in many foods.

## Caloric Content

Inulin is broken down in the colon. It provides 1 ½ calories per gram, making it a popular substitute for sugars and fats.
Sugar contains four calories per gram and fat contains nine calories per gram.

## Use in Foods

When inulin is sheared with water or milk, micro-crystals are formed to create a smooth, creamy, fat-like feel in the mouth. Because of its low caloric content, sweet taste and fat-like feel, inulin is very popular in diet foods.

## Inulin in Processed Foods—Man-made Inulin—Not Good!

Inulin is increasingly used in processed foods because it has unusually adaptable characteristics. Its flavor ranges from bland to subtly sweet (approx. 10% sweetness of sugar/sucrose). It can be used to replace sugar, fat, and flour.

Fructans are chains of fructose and wheat has fructans in it therefore making it unsuitable for many who have Fructose Malabsorption General Diet Information listed as an example:

A fructan is a polymer of fructose molecules. Fructans with a short chain length are known as fructooligosaccharides, whereas longer chain fructans are termed inulins.

Fructans occur in foods such as agave, artichokes, asparagus, leeks, garlic, onions (including spring onions), and wheat.

In animal fodder, fructans also appear in grass, with dietary implications for horses and other Equidae.

Take time to understand how Fructans and Fructans Inulin-type play a part in your digestive system.

Inulin-type fructans are non-digestible; they are fermented in the colon, and classified as dietary fiber and prebiotic.

The fermentation produces large amounts of gas, often resulting in bloating, flatulence and abdominal pain or cramps.

Remember Inulin is Another Word for Fructose!

Animal and emerging human research have demonstrated the following inulin effects: modification of composition and activities of the gut flora, improved stool production, enhanced absorption of calcium and other minerals, regulation of gastrointestinal endocrine peptides, increased immunity and resistance to infections, improved lipid homeostasis.

Fructans as listed below is why anyone that Hereditary Fructose Intolerance or Malabsorption can't eat these foods they will produce the symptoms and pain after ingesting them. Fructans are a form of dietary fiber. However, these foods will produce pain and inflammation to HFI or FM individuals after ingesting them.

They consist of linked molecules of the sugar fructose and a lesser number of glucose molecules. Many forms of fructans exist in a variety of vegetables, grains, and fruit.

## Healthy Digestive System

Inulin is a prebiotic. Prebiotics serve as foods for probiotics, which helps maintain a healthy digestive system.

Inulin is a polysaccharide that is produced by plants such as onions, leeks, Jerusalem artichokes, and garlic. It can also be referred to as neosugar, alant starch, Alantin, and diabetic sugar.

It can also be used to replace higher calorie ingredients such as fat, sugar, and flour. However, there is also some controversy about how much it should be used.

When eaten, this substance does not increase blood sugar, which makes it an option for those with diabetes.

It has one-third to one-fourth less food energy than that of sugar and a sixth to a ninth less energy than fat. It is also a soluble fiber, which means that when it passes through the body, it creates a gel. Since fiber is not digested in the human body, it passes through to the intestine largely intact. There, it feeds the good bacteria that live there. It also helps to reduce the absorption of bad cholesterol in the body.

This allows the bacteria that feed on them to thrive and increase intestinal function.

It should be noted that too much can produce bloating, gas, diarrhea, and other symptoms in some people. This is especially true for those who are sensitive to the substance.

Some denounce the use of refined inulin as an additive to food. These opponents argue that refining one substance out of its food context can cause more harm than good.

They cite the fact that the substance doesn't just encourage the growth of good bacteria but can also feed certain yeasts found in the intestine. It can also feed bad bacteria such as klebsiella.

I don't think inulin is good when it's not in its natural form and I agree with the article that it can do more harm than good if we consume too much of it.

Conversely, it is also considered a class of carbohydrates, which are problematic for some individuals through causing overgrowth of intestinal (SIBO or IBS) methanogenic bacteria.

The consumption of large quantities (in particular, by sensitive or unaccustomed individuals) can lead to gas and bloating, and products that contain inulin will sometimes include a warning to add it gradually to one's diet.

Due to the body's limited ability to process fructans, inulin has minimal increasing impact on blood sugar. It is considered suitable for diabetics and potentially helpful in managing blood sugar-related illness.

The intolerance often only becomes apparent in adulthood.

This common and benign form of fructose intolerance must be distinguished from the rare and potentially dangerous hereditary fructose intolerance (HFI).

Fructose consumption has increased markedly in the last few decades and is implicated in the rapid increase in childhood obesity, the metabolic syndrome, and certain liver disease and much more!

## Frequency in Population and Natural History

- Approximately 30% of healthy adults show malabsorption of fructose doses below 50g, but less than 10% have symptomatic intolerance. There appear to be no major racial differences.
- Up to 65% of patients with Irritable Bowel Syndrome have fructose intolerance due to malabsorption.
- Commonly appears in adults and may be triggered by stress or inflammation.

Currently, I see many probiotics on the market and they are suppose to be the most current and highly developed products produced by our pharmaceutical companies, their target audience is toward the Irritable Bowel Syndrome individual.

They tell you that it will help with your bloating, diarrhea, constipation, and IBS symptoms. It is a step in the right direction but the doctors and pharmaceutical companies are singing the same old tune. Take this new "Pill" and it will make you feel better.

They market their products toward the damaged intestinal flora knowing that their product alone can't fix our digestive problems without first changing our diets! Ultimately, we gain nothing but an added expense. These companies once again are providing a counterproductive product. Only when you eradicate the foods that create the problems will your health return.

## Prebiotic: (33)

Prebiotics are non-digestible food ingredients that stimulate the growth and/or activity of bacteria in the digestive system in ways claimed to be beneficial to health.

## Probiotics: (33)

Probiotics are live bacteria that may confer a health benefit on the host. In the past, there were other definitions of probiotics.

Probiotics is described as "live microbial feed supplement which beneficially affects the host animal by improving its intestinal microbial balance."

Through 2012, however, in all cases proposed as health claims to the European Food Safety Authority, the scientific evidence remains insufficient to prove a cause and effect relationship between consumption of probiotic products and any health benefit.

When a person takes antibiotics, both the harmful bacteria and the beneficial bacteria are killed. A reduction of beneficial bacteria can lead to digestive problems, such as diarrhea, yeast infections, and urinary tract infections. The possibility that supplemental probiotics affect such digestive issues is unknown, and remains under study.

## Sorbitol---Yet, another Concern!

What else do you need to look for in our modern diet? Sorbitol and xylitol (polyol) intolerances

Sorbitol and xylitol consumption should be reduced to a minimum, due to the high degree of concurrent intolerance and symptom exacerbation (see Sorbitol intolerance).

Food allergies may co-exist with sugar intolerances. Generally, telltale signs of possible additional allergies are skin rashes and itching, sinusitis or asthma and hay fever.

Lactose and fructose intolerance co-exist in approximately 20-30% of individuals.

Sorbitol, xylitol, and fructose intolerances very commonly co-exist and may exacerbate each other (see Sorbitol intolerance***).

Sorbitol is a sugar alcohol what doctors call a polyol commonly used as a sweetener in sugar-free sweets and chewing gum, diet, and diabetic foods, amongst other products.

It is produced by the human body, occurs in fruit, beer and berries, is also contained in some medicines (e.g. mouthwashes, cough syrups, and laxatives) and cosmetics.

Absorption in the small intestine occurs passively and is much slower than other sugars.

This allows even moderate doses to be malabsorbed, reaching the colon for fermentation, especially in individuals with a rapid intestinal transit.

A high proportion of healthy individuals develop abdominal bloating, gas, cramps, and diarrhea at doses of 5 g and above.

Fructose and sorbitol intolerance often co-exist and mutually aggravate intestinal symptoms.

The concurrence of lactose and sorbitol is less clear, although there is some supporting evidence (see Lactose intolerance).

## Frequency in Population

More than 50% of adults experience significant symptoms following ingestion of more than 10 g.

Present in up to 65% of patients with Irritable Bowel Syndrome also had malabsorbed Sorbitol.

## Symptoms

These include bloating, abdominal cramps and pain, diarrhea, increased intestinal sounds and gas production, and nausea. These symptoms resemble those of functional bowel disease. Up to 70% of patients with irritable bowel syndrome are sorbitol intolerant.

Little is known about long term effects of sorbitol intolerance, although severe weight loss has been reported.

In diabetics, high concentrations of sorbitol secondary to high blood glucose concentrations have been associated with nerve (small nerve fiber neuropathy) as well as eye damage.

## Management

Reduction of the intake of sorbitol to individually tolerated levels will rapidly lead to symptom relief in most individuals.

Sorbitol is frequently encountered in diet, i.e. low calorie, foods and beverages, in high concentrations in sugar-free chewing gum and sweets / candies, in stone fruit (e.g. sweet cherries, plums) and dried fruit. Liquid medicines may contain sorbitol.

Fructose intolerance should be excluded by appropriate testing, due to the high degree of concurrent intolerance and symptom exacerbation.

Every Diagnosis I have listed in my book has symptoms that you can cross-reference with those of a Fructose Malabsorption health issue. I'm sure this is not a coincidence. I'm sure we don't want to risk our health or the health of our family by allowing HFCS to remain in our diets. That is why I am an advocate of organic foods and shop at Whole Foods.

Many people may have doubts...but I have lived through this nightmare and I stand as living proof that HFCS can decimate your health. I can also substantiate that a diet that is comprised of fresh organic food can heal my body, both physically and mentally.

What part of your body do you want to put at risk?

If you are serious about improving your health while lessening your bowel distress, I highly recommended changes be made to your existing diet immediately. It was crucial in reclaiming my digestive health to find out what I could and could not eat. Understanding your body and what fuel it needs to run at maximum capacity is vital for your continued existence.

Everyone who has any of the diagnoses I have listed which are, Irritable Bowel Syndrome, Gluten, Lactose, Celiac, Polyol, Fructose Malabsorption or HFI, Leaky Gut, Crohn's, Colitis, and SIBO will benefit from this chapter. All of the diseases are linked to what you eat!

People who follow a more natural diet low in processed foods eat about 60% of their foods fresh and uncooked, thereby receiving the maximum benefits provided by antioxidants and soluble fibres found in fruits and vegetables. These benefits include improved digestive health, cancer reductions, and prevention of diverticulosis.

I created the Fructose-Specific Food Charts...especially for Fructose challenged individuals.

Some diet suggestions are devoid of manufactured foods - thus letting you eat as past generations did before the advent of commercialism overrunning our kitchens.

My Fructose-Specific Food Charts assists you in returning to very modest fructose consumption - that is, only fructose naturally found in fruits and vegetables. It would be very difficult, by consuming fructose found only in fruits and vegetables, to exceed 20 grams per day, thereby staying well below the limit that causes fructose malabsorption problems.

For people who are very fructose-sensitive, high-fructose foods may create huge problems - but are easy to avoid.

In a paper published by Dr. Rao of Augusta, Georgia investigating the long-term impact of a fructose-restricted diet on digestive symptoms in fructose-intolerant patients - over half of the patients were able to remain compliant with their diet over a 12-month period. (34)

This group reported a significant improvement in their symptoms of abdominal pain, fullness, indigestion, and diarrhea.

It is important for people to be properly diagnosed for fructose malabsorption since the necessary dietary modifications are a challenge to apply and require a lifelong commitment. Despite the challenges, the halt of bowel symptoms can provide positive reinforcement in remaining faithful to a diet regimen. Dietary lapses are not harmful (unless you have been diagnosed with a Hereditary form) rather they provide strong reminders of why you are on the diet!

It needs to be emphasized that success with a fructose-restricted diet is best achieved through education. That is the main reason I have gone into such detail on what you can or what you can't eat...and the impact of the foods or lack of vitamins and minerals due to a high fructose diet.

For continued success, us my Fructose-Specific Food Charts, as well as, the support of your family and Friends. Your family needs to make the changes with you.

Studies have shown that for those who heed and manage dietary modifications and restrictions, bowel symptoms are significantly improved and sustained for years.

## A Calorie Has Never Been Just a Calorie

Calories must be looked at and compared to the type of calorie it is...i.e. is it coming from fat or sugar etc. Glucose is the form of energy you were designed to run on. Every cell in your body, every bacterium...in fact, every living thing on the Earth uses glucose for energy.

If you received your fructose from only fruits and vegetables (where it originates) as most people did a century ago, you'd consume just a few grams a day and it is certainly a huge difference in the approximate 100 to 150 grams per day that the average adolescent gets from sweetened drinks.

In vegetables and fruits, fructose is mixed with fiber, vitamins, minerals, enzymes all that moderate any negative metabolic effects.

Your body metabolizes fructose in a much different way than glucose. The entire burden of metabolizing fructose falls on your liver. People are consuming fructose in enormous quantities, which has made the negative effects that more profound.

Yet as the low-fat craze spread, rates of heart disease, diabetes, and obesity skyrocketed...clearly, this plan was seriously flawed from the get-go, and it's not difficult to see that trading fat for sugar and chemicals is not a wise move.

Without a doubt, we now know that excessive fructose content in the modern diet that is taking a devastating toll on people's health.

There are too few doctors and/or hospitals currently researching this issue...education must me increased now!

At the heart of it, all is the fact that excessive fructose consumption leads to insulin resistance, and insulin resistance appears to be the root of many if not most chronic disease. Insulin resistance has even been found to be an underlying factor of cancer.

How High Fructose Corn Syrup has and is Decimating Human Health.

Food and beverage manufacturers quickly began switching their sweeteners from sucrose (table sugar) to corn syrup when they discovered that it could save them a lot of money. Sucrose costs about three times as much as HFCS. HFCS is also about 20 percent sweeter than table sugar, so you need less to achieve the same amount of sweetness.

Around that same time, dietary fats were blamed for heart disease, giving rise to the "low-fat craze," which resulted in an explosion of processed nonfat and low fat convenience foods—most of which tasted like sawdust unless sugar was added. Fructose was then added to make all these fat-free products more palatable.

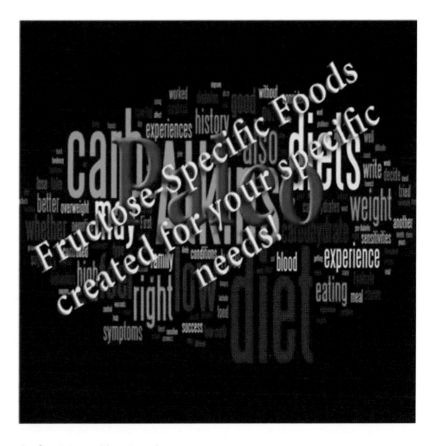

Carbs: Never Too Low!

Dietary carbs, such as sugars and starches are not needed, because the liver can convert fat and protein into glucose.

Thus, diabetics, who have a hard time balancing their dietary intake of carbs with the insulin that they inject, can simplify the process by routinely eating less carbs spread through many meals and triggering some glucose production by the liver.

Craving for carbohydrates/sweets can be dramatically reduced simply by eating fewer carbs and avoiding insulin production that can lead to more dramatic swings of blood sugars and hunger. Using this strategy, you will be hungry less than once a week.

If you plan what you are going to eat and you pre-prepare your foods you will be able to grab a "quick" fix from the fridge instead of eating something you will regret. You will find you can break the "Sugar" bad "Carbohydrate" cycle!

## How Much Fructose Are You Consuming?

It's no secret that we are eating more sugar than at any other time in history. In 1700, the average person ate very little sugar within a day's time.

Today, a large percent of all Americans consume over 134 grams of fructose a day, according to research. That kind of consumption equates to more than 100 pounds of sugar per year!

It just so happens that this statistic dovetails nicely with the statistics showing that one in four Americans is either pre-diabetic or has type II diabetes Fructose seems to be at the root of many type II diabetes issues.

As a standard recommendation, I strongly advise keeping your TOTAL fructose consumption below 20 grams per day

For most people it would actually be wise to limit your fruit fructose to 15 grams or less, as you're virtually guaranteed to get "hidden" fructose from just about any processed food you might eat, including condiments you might never have suspected would contain sugar.

Keep in mind that fruits also contain fructose, although an ameliorating factor is that whole fruits also contain vitamins and other antioxidants that reduce the hazardous effects of fructose.

Again, one way to determine just how strict you need to be is to check your uric acid levels. If you feel strongly that fruits are exceptionally beneficial to you and don't believe this recommendation then at least test your uric acid level.

Consume whatever level of fructose and fruits you believe is healthy for a few days and then have your uric acid level measured.

If it is outside the healthy ranges listed above, then I strongly suggest you listen to your body's biochemical feedback and reduce your fructose consumption until your uric acid levels normalize.

Juices are nearly as detrimental as soda, because a glass of juice is loaded with fructose, and many of the antioxidants are lost.

It isn't as simple as merely selecting and eating fresh foods. You must know how anything your digest is absorbed. Understanding why a particular food has a negative impact on you is important in order for you not to suffer from Fructose Malabsorption.

Selecting healthy foods is an education for all of us!

## Fructose-Specific Food Charts

To assure you that I have tested the foods in my charts I wanted to break down the Fructose level of an Apple. This will allow you to understand why your body may not be able digest it properly. All foods listed on my charts have been tested and I have used this method as support my findings for my Fructose-Specific Food.

I use the Fineli Chart (this Chart can be downloaded to your smart phone) for quick reference when needed

If an apple has a total sugar count of 8.1 grams, you need to break it down in this manner.

Total Sucrose (remember this is equal parts of Glucose and Fructose):          2.4 G

Total Fructose:          4.3 G

Total Glucose:          1.4 G

What is the total fructose for this food type? It is 5.5 grams of fructose to only 1.4 grams of glucose so the small intestine (if you have fructose malabsorption or hereditary fructose intolerance you would find this difficult to digest.

The fructose far outweighs the glucose. You need to look at the sucrose level and divide it by 2, then add that percentage to the fructose level listed which is 4.3.   Half of the 2.4 g of sucrose is 1.2 grams and once you add that additional fructose to your total you have a food that people with FM or HFI can't digest properly without consequences.

Glucose is needed in order to process fructose – so glucose (or dextrose) is good.

When balancing a fructose diet you must look for items that have a higher level of glucose in them then fructose and unfortunately, this is not general knowledge and takes a great deal of time to track down the correct items. This is why I created my own Food Chart and I will continually fine-tune the charts.

Note: Research has shown that HFCS to be a leading factor in health decline! (35)

One of the primary sources of HFCS in the American diet is soda – in fact, many public health advocates refer to soda as "liquid candy." That nickname is more apt than advocates realized, according to a study published online this month by the journal Obesity.

The HFCS used in soda is supposed to contain no more than 55% fructose and 45% glucose, according to the Corn Refiners Assn. (Another popular formulation is 42% fructose and 58% glucose.) This slight difference (and I believe inaccurate percentage) is the reason why we frequently say that HFCS is just as unhealthy as "natural" sugar.

However, it turns out that some of the stuff they put in soda isn't HFCS, it's RHFCS – Really High Fructose Corn Syrup.

The Keck researchers found that the sweeteners in Coca-Cola and Pepsi contained as much as 65% fructose (and only 35% glucose), and Sprite registered as much as 64% fructose (and 36% glucose). (35)

"The type of sugar listed on the label is not always consistent with the type of sugar detected," they wrote.

"Considering that the average American drinks 50 gallons of soda and other sweetened beverages each year, it is important that we have more precise information regarding what they contain, including a listing of the fructose content." (35)

HFCS or Corn Syrup is in everything these days! It is in our Hot Dogs, Soda, Vitamin Water, Sports Drinks, Tea Bags (yes in some Tea Bags) all Fast Food items and is used heavily in…Bakery Items, Bread, Peanut Butter, Buns, Canned Food, Pre-packaged and Frozen foods…did you really think using any food item with this substance in it was going to keep you "SLIM AND HEALTHY"?

Look around to see how many people look slim while devouring their extra large diet soda, fast food or zero calorie no-fat foods!

## Acidity Factor in Your Diet!

Various foods contain acids or alkalis and other foods create acidity or alkalinity in the body when combined with juices and digestive acids. A diet rich in alkali-forming foods is important to ongoing good health. It assists with detoxification, as the body is already working to remove the acidic waste products of metabolism you certainly don't want to add to the burden.

I read during my research that the level of acid within your body is slightly more alkaline than neutral. You can actually test this at home using litmus paper strips to test your saliva. You can purchase these strips on line or at a vitamin store.

The health implications of our acidic lives are currently being seen in the loss of bone density. More and more women are being diagnosed with osteoporosis. Many physicians will suggest a calcium supplement for their patients to get bone-building calcium. However, calcium is not deposited in the bones without adequate levels of vitamin D, yet few physicians test vitamin D levels. If doctors would follow a protocol by checking the toxicity and acidic conditions, first…the patient would be on a life-improvement track to good health in which the body could reverse the harmful effects. In addition, could prevent a life-harming protocol.

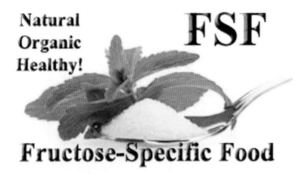

**Natural Organic Healthy!** **FSF**

**Fructose-Specific Food**

As you select and fine-tune "your" foods, take in account that on an average it takes 3 days for an overconsumption of Fructose to go through you body. This period is based on my own research as I gathered information on what I could and couldn't eat. I'm very sensitive to fructose so keep that in mind.

Only add a new food item every 4 to 5 days so you can be sure of how your body reacts. Fructose-Specific Food Charts were created by Nancie Paruso for my own personal use. This is the only chart that is created specifically for Fructose issues.

My weight went from 164 is 112, my energy is high, and I have no depression and the pain has diminished by 90 to 95% of what it was. It does take some planning for meals but it is doable. In the beginning, you can simplify your life by creating a weekly menu planner.

Once you have eliminated a large portion of Fructose from your diet you will feel better, and you will have learned what you can and can't have. A food planner is simply a tool I use to I know what impacts me in a negative manner and how long it takes the fructose to be out of my system. Ultimately, it is your decision

| Food Item | Tolerated | CT= Can't Tolerate HFI individuals can't tolerate but FM may be able to tolerate | May be able to tolerate in small doses | Harvard Medical | Boston University Diet for HFI | Mayo Clinic | Univ. Iowa |
|---|---|---|---|---|---|---|---|
| Alfalfa | X | X HFI | | | X | X | |
| All Deserts Containing Honey | | X HFI | | X | X | X | |
| All Deserts Containing Sugar | | X HFI | **X** | X | X | X | |
| All hard Cheese | X | X HFI | | X | X | X | |
| Any other processed meat | | X | | X | X | X | |
| Apple Juice | | X | | X | | X | |
| Apple/Dried | | X | | X | | X | X |
| Apples Raw | | X | | X | | X | X |
| Apricots/Raw | | X | | X | | X | X |
| Artichoke depends on type | X | X HFI | | X | X | X | X |
| Artichoke Globe | | X | | X | | X | X |
| Artichoke Jerusalem | | X | | X | | X | X |
| Asparagus | X HFI | X | | X | X | X | X |
| Avocado | X Iowa | | | | | | X |
| Bacon | | X | | X | X | X | X |

All agreed not for HFI

184

| Food Item | Tolerated | CT= Can't Tolerate HFI individuals can't tolerate but FM may be able to tolerate | May be able to tolerate in small doses | Harvard Medical | Boston University Diet for HFI | Mayo Clinic | Univ. Iowa |
|---|---|---|---|---|---|---|---|
| Baked Beans | | X | | X | X | X | X |
| Baked potatoes | X | | | X | | X | X |
| Bamboo Shoots | X | | | | X | X | |
| Banana (if not over-ripe) Has fructose but has more Glucose so the body can break it down properly. | X | | | X | | X | X |
| Basil | X | | | X | | X | X |
| Bean Shoots | X | | | X | | X | X |
| Beef | X | | | X | X | X | X |
| Beef Pattie no bread or condiments | X | | | | | | X |
| Beets | | X | | X | X | X | X |
| Bell Pepper | X | | X per H&M | X | | X | |
| Blackberry | | X | | X | | X | X |
| Blueberries | X | | X | | | | X |
| Boysenberries | X | | | X | | X | X |
| Bread check labels no sugar or high fructose corn syrup(no bread, crackers or saltines) | | XHFI | | X | X | | X |

| Food Item | Tolerated | CT= Can't Tolerate HFI individuals can't tolerate but FM may be able to tolerate | May be able to tolerate in small doses | Harvard Medical | Boston University Diet for HFI | Mayo Clinic | Univ. Iowa |
|---|---|---|---|---|---|---|---|
| Broccoli | | X | | X | | X | X |
| Brussels Sprouts | | X | X | | | X | X |
| Butter | XHFI | | | X | X | X | X |
| Cabbage | | X | X HFI | X | X | X | X |
| Canned Fruit | | X | | X | X | X | X |
| Cantaloupe | X | | | | X | X | X |
| Carbonated Beverages | | XHFI | | X | X | X | X |
| Carmel | | X | | X | X | X | X |
| Carob powder | | X | | X | | X | X |
| Carrots | X | X HFI | X Per H&M | X | X | X | X |
| Catsup | | XHFI | | X | X | X | X |
| Cauliflower | X | X | X Per H&M | X | X | X | X |
| Caution no over-ripe fruits | X | X | X | X | | X | X |
| Celery | X | | | X | X | X | X |
| Cereal (no cereal with sugar added) | | X | | X | X | X | X |
| Cherries (sweet) | | X | | X | X | X | X |
| Chervil per U of Iowa | | X | | | | | X |
| Chick Peas | X IOWA | X | | X | X | X | X |
| Chicken | X | | | X | X | X | X |
| Chicory (coffee substitutes) | | X | | X | X | X | X |
| Chicory Roots | | X | | X | X | X | X |
| Chili Powder | | X | | X | X | X | X |

| Food Item | Tolerated | CT = Can't Tolerate HFI individuals can't tolerate but FM may be able to tolerate | May be able to tolerate in small doses | Harvard Medical | Boston University Diet for HFI | Mayo Clinic | Univ. Iowa |
|---|---|---|---|---|---|---|---|
| Chili Sauce | | XHFI | | | X | | X |
| Chives | X IOWA | | | | | | X |
| Choko | X | X HFI | | X | X | X | X |
| Choy | X | X HFI | | X | X | X | X |
| Choy Sum | X | X HFI | | X | X | X | X |
| Cinnamon | XHFI | X Per H&M | | X | X | X | X |
| Coffee | XHFI | | | X | X | X | X |
| Compotes (canned fruits and Syrup) | | X | | X | X | X | X |
| Cookies | | X | | X | X | X | X |
| Coriander | X | X IOWA | | | X | X | X |
| Corn | | X | | X | X | X | X |
| Couscous | | X | | X | X | X | X |
| Crackers | | X | | X | X | X | X |
| Cranberries Note: Tolerance may be dose dependent per U of I | X | | | | X | | X |
| Dandelion Greens | X IOWA | X | | X | X | X | X |
| Dates | | X | | X | X | X | X |
| Dill weed | | X IOWA | | | | | X |
| Dried apples | | X | | X | X | X | X |
| Dried currants | | X | | X | X | X | X |
| Dried dates | | X | | X | X | X | X |
| Dried figs | | X | | X | X | X | X |
| Dried pears | | X | | X | X | X | X |

187

| Food Item | Tolerated | CT= Can't Tolerate HFI individuals can't tolerate but FM may be able to tolerate | May be able to tolerate in small doses | Harvard Medical | Boston University Diet for HFI | Mayo Clinic | Univ. Iowa |
|---|---|---|---|---|---|---|---|
| Egg Plant | | X | | X | X | X | X |
| Eggs | X | | | X | X | X | X |
| Endive | X | X HFI | | X | X | X | X |
| Escarole Note: Tolerance maybe dose dependent | X IOWA | | | | | | X |
| Fennel | | X | X IOWA | | X | X | X |
| Figs | | X | | X | X | X | X |
| Fish | X | | | X | X | X | X |
| Fresh Potatoes not canned or Frozen | X | | | X | X | X | X |
| Frozen Fruit | | X | | X | X | X | X |
| Fruit compotes | | X | | X | X | X | X |
| Fruit juice | | X | | X | X | X | X |
| Fruit juice concentrates | | X | | X | X | X | X |
| Garlic | | XHFI FOR ALL FM PER IOWA | | | X | | X |
| Gelato | X | | | | X | | |
| Ginger | X | X HFI X IOWA | X H&M | X | X | X | X |
| Gluten-free bread or cereal products | X | | | X | X | X | X |
| Grape Juice (White) | | X | | X | X | X | X |
| Grapefruit | X | | | | X | X | X |
| Grapes | | X | | X | X | X | X |

| Food Item | Tolerated | CT= Can't Tolerate HFI individuals can't tolerate but FM may be able to tolerate | May be able to tolerate in small doses | Harvard Medical | Boston University Diet for HFI | Mayo Clinic | Univ. Iowa |
|---|---|---|---|---|---|---|---|
| Green Beans | X | | | X | X | X | X |
| Green Peas | | X | | X | X | X | X |
| Green Peppers | X | | | X | X | X | X |
| Guava | | X | | X | | X | X |
| Gum | | X HFI | | X | X | X | X |
| Ham | | X | | X | X | X | X |
| Hard cheeses | X | | | X | X | X | X |
| Homemade French Dressing No Sugar | X HFI | | | | X | | X |
| Homemade Mayonnaise No Sugar | X HFI | | | | X | | X |
| Honey Melon | | X | | X | X | X | X |
| Honeydew Melon | | X | | X | X | X | X |
| Hot Dogs | | X HFI | | X | X | X | X |
| Hydrogenated starch hydrolysates HSH | | X | | X | X | X | X |
| Iceberg Lettuce | | X | | | X | X | X |
| Jam | | X HFI | | X | X | X | X |
| Jellies | | X | | X | X | X | X |
| Kaki | | X | | | X | | |
| Kidney Beans | | X | | X | X | X | X |
| KIWI | | X | | X | | X | X |
| Lactose Free Yogurt | X | | X H&M | X | | X | |
| Lactose-free milk | X | | | | | X | |

| Food Item | Tolerated | CT= Can't Tolerate HFI individuals can't tolerate but FM may be able to tolerate | May be able to tolerate in small doses | Harvard Medical | Boston University Diet for HFI | Mayo Clinic | Univ. Iowa |
|---|---|---|---|---|---|---|---|
| Lamb | X | | | X | X | X | |
| Leeks | | X | | X | X | X | X |
| Lemongrass | X | | | | X | | |
| Lentils | X IOWA | | | | | | X |
| Licorice | | X | | X | X | | |
| Lima Beans | X IOWA | | | | | | X |
| Litese | | X | | | X | | X |
| Low Calorie Foods and Soft Drinks | | X | | X | X | X | X |
| Lunch Meats | | X | | X | X | X | X |
| Macaroni | X HFI | | | X | X | X | X |
| Mango | | X | | X | X | X | X |
| Marjoram | X | | | X | | | X |
| Milk  *** Check for additives NO SWEETENED | X | | | X | X | X | X |
| Mint Flavor | X | | | X | | | X |
| Mints | | X HFI | | X | X | X | X |
| Mung Beans | X IOWA | | | | | | X |
| Mushrooms | X IOWA | | | | | | X |
| Mustard Greens | X IOWA | | | | | | X |
| Nashi Fruit | | X | | X | | | X |

| Food Item | Tolerated | CT= Can't Tolerate HFI individuals can't tolerate but FM may be able to tolerate | May be able to tolerate in small doses | Harvard Medical | Boston University Diet for HFI | Mayo Clinic | Univ. Iowa |
|---|---|---|---|---|---|---|---|
| New White Potatoes (Canned) | | X | | X | X | X | X |
| No Fruits | | XHFI | X FODMAP & BOSTON U | X | X | X | X |
| No Sugar | | X | | | | | X |
| Noodles | X HFI | | | X | X | X | X |
| Nuts other than Pistachios | X IOWA | | | | | | X |
| Nuts Pistachios 2 or 3 Tbsp | X IOWA | | | | | | X |
| Oats | X | | | X | | X | X |
| Oil Canola | | XHFI | | X | X | X | X |
| Okra | | X | | X | X | X | X |
| Olive Oil | X | | | X | | | X |
| Olives | X | X HFI | | X | X | X | X |
| Onions | | X HFI | | X | X | X | X |
| Onions, Spring Onions | | X | | X | X | X | X |
| Orange | | X | Unclear | | | | X |
| Orange Juice | | X | | X | X | X | X |
| Organic Butter | X | | | X | X | X | X |
| Papaya | | X | | X | | X | X |
| Parsley | X | X Iowa | | X | | X | X |
| Parsnip | X | X HFI | | X | X | X | X |
| Pasta no red sauce | | | X | | | | X |
| Pawpaw | | X | | X | X | X | X |
| Peaches/Raw | | X | | X | X | X | X |
| Peaches/Dried | | X | | X | X | X | X |

| Food Item | Tolerated | CT= Can't Tolerate HFI individuals can't tolerate but FM may be able to tolerate | May be able to tolerate in small doses | Harvard Medical | Boston University Diet for HFI | Mayo Clinic | Univ. Iowa |
|---|---|---|---|---|---|---|---|
| Pear Juice | | X | | X | X | X | X |
| Pears Raw | | X | | X | X | X | X |
| Pepper | X HFI | | | X | X | X | X |
| Pineapple* | | X | | X | X | X | X |
| Plums Raw | | X | | X | X | X | X |
| Polenta | X | | | | | | X |
| Pomegranate | | X | | X | X | | X |
| Pork | X | | | X | X | X | X |
| Prune Juice | | | X | | X | X | X |
| Prunes | | | X | | X | X | X |
| Pumpkin | X | | | X | X | X | X |
| Pumpkin Pie Seasonings | | X IOWA | | | | | X |
| Quince | | X | | X | | X | X |
| Raisin | | X | | X | | X | X |
| Raspberries see notes | X | | | X | | X | X |
| Red Capsicum | X | X HFI | | | X | | |
| Rice | X HFI | | | X | X | X | |
| Rice Milk | X | | | | X | | |
| Romaine Lettuce | X | | | X | X | X | X |
| Roman lettuce with mushrooms hard cheese oil/balsamic vinegar | X | | | | | | X |
| Rosemary | X | | | X | X | X | |
| Rye Bread without High Fructose Corn Syrup | X | Rye Bread must be mad from rye flour | | | | X | X |

192

| Food Item | Tolerated | CT= Can't Tolerate HFI individuals can't tolerate but FM may be able to tolerate | May be able to tolerate in small doses | Harvard Medical | Boston University Diet for HFI | Mayo Clinic | Univ. Iowa |
|---|---|---|---|---|---|---|---|
| Rye Whole Meal Bread | | X | | X | | | |
| Salt | X HFI | | | X | X | X | X |
| Sede | X | X HFI | | | X | | |
| Shallots | X HFI | | | X | X | X | X |
| Silver Beet | X | X HFI | | | X | | |
| Sorbet | X | | | | | | X |
| Soy Milk | X | | | X | | | X |
| Spelt Bread 100% | | X | | X | | | |
| Spinach | X | | | X | X | X | X |
| Star Fruit | | X | | X | X | X | X |
| Strawberries has glucose and fiber to break this down properly See Notes | X | | X HFI | X | X | X | X |
| Sugar Free Chewing Gum | | X | X HFI | X | | X | X |
| Summer Squash | X | | | X | X | X | X |
| Swede | | X | | | X | | |
| Sweet Corn | | X | | X | X | X | X |
| Sweet Potato | | X HFI | | X | X | X | X |
| Sweet Potatoes in skin, boiled | | X | | X | X | X | X |

| Food Item | Tolerated | CT = Can't Tolerate HFI individuals can't tolerate but FM may be able to tolerate | May be able to tolerate in small doses | Harvard Medical | Boston University Diet for HFI | Mayo Clinic | Univ. Iowa |
|---|---|---|---|---|---|---|---|
| Swiss Chard | X IOWA | | | | | | X |
| Taro | X | X HFI | | | X | | |
| Tea | X HFI | | | X | X | X | X |
| Thyme | X | | | X | X | X | X |
| Tomato | X | X HFI | | X | X | X | X |
| Tortilla wrap with sliced beef | X | | | | | | X |
| Turkey | X | | | X | X | X | X |
| Turnip | X | X HFI  X IOWA | | X | X | X | X |
| Turnip Greens | X IOWA | | | | | | X |
| Veal | X | | | X | X | X | X |
| Vitamin and Medication Syrups (for Children) | | | X | | X | | |
| Watermelon | | X | | | X | | |
| Wax Beans | X | X HFI | | | X | | |
| Wheat (Bread Pasta, Pastry) Check Sugar | | X | | X | X | | |
| White Potato Fresh Only | X HFI | | | | X | | |
| Whole Wheat | | X | | X | X | X | X |

| Food Item | Tolerated | CT= Can't Tolerate HFI individuals can't tolerate but FM may be able to tolerate | May be able to tolerate in small doses | Harvard Medical | Boston University Diet for HFI | Mayo Clinic | Univ. Iowa |
|---|---|---|---|---|---|---|---|
| Yam | X | X HFI | | | X | | |
| Yellow Potatoes | | X | | X | X | X | X |
| Zucchini | X | | | | X | | |

I strongly suggest that if you don't or can't buy organic than at least buy "Fresh" foods.

This will make a big change in your health…most grocery stores now have an organic section…so if you don't have an organic store near you…look for this section in your store or try going to a local "Farmers" market.

I know that Publix and Fresh Market carry organic food and I shop at both but Whole Foods is the best for everything you need ORGANIC"! We now have a Whole Foods in my town.

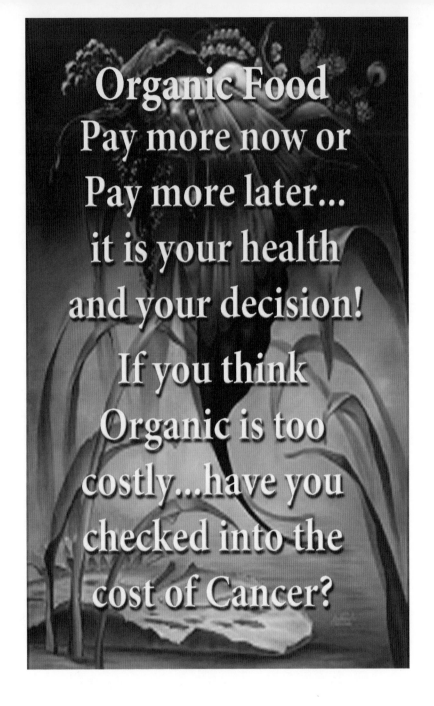

Organic Food
Pay more now or
Pay more later...
it is your health
and your decision!

If you think
Organic is too
costly...have you
checked into the
cost of Cancer?

If you can't eat Organic...please eat Fresh!

## Healthfulness of Sweeteners

--From Most Healthy...To Least Healthy--AGE

This is rating the sweeteners from safest, Stevia to most unhealthy/dangerous fructose/agave syrup.

- Stevia - is a protein that is sweet, doesn't raise blood sugar, no insulin spike and no AGE
- Glucose - raises blood sugar, spikes insulin and produces AGE
- Xylitol - is a sugar alcohol that inhibits dental bacteria, doesn't raise blood sugar, no
- insulin spike or AGE
- Corn Syrup - raises blood sugar, spikes insulin, produces AGE, low sweetness
- Sucrose - raises blood sugar, spikes insulin and produces AGE, and liver damage
- Honey - is half fructose and half glucose, raises blood sugar, spikes insulin, produces high
- AGE and may damage liver
- Artificial Sweeteners, aspartame, sucralose, saccharin, etc. - don't raise blood sugar or
- produce AGE (***SEE NOTE***) but may have other risks, including hunger
- HFCS - is high fructose corn syrup, raises blood sugar and spikes insulin, produces very high AGE and causes liver damage
- Fructose - doesn't raise blood sugar or spike insulin, produces very high AGE and causes liver damage
- Agave Nectar - is fructose, doesn't raise blood sugar or spike insulin, produces very high AGE and causes liver damage

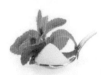

# FIND OUT WHAT WORKS FOR YOU!

I have found there are substitutes for those times when I crave something sweet...I eat fresh fruit that is on my approved list and I have found that for "me" stevia is a good substitute as a sweetener for my coffee and tea.

Recently a new sweetener was put on the market. This was in direct competition with the current Stevia market. It is made from a natural fruit and it is zero calories.

What they are not telling you is that "Monk" fruit is notable for its sweetness, which can be concentrated from its juice. The fruit contains 25 to 38% of various carbohydrates, mainly <u>fructose and glucose. The sweetness of this fruit is increased by the mogrosides</u>, a group of triterpene glycosides (saponins). If a natural fruit has too much Fructose in its composition...it is going to be a problem for your digestive tract.

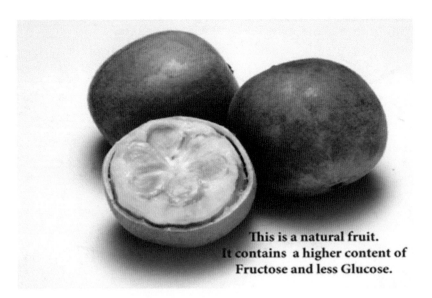

**This is a natural fruit.
It contains a higher content of
Fructose and less Glucose.**

| Food Item | Tolerated | CT = Can't Tolerate / HFI individuals can't tolerate but FM may be able to tolerate | May be able to tolerate in small doses | Harvard Medical | Boston University Article/FODMAP | Mayo Clinic | Univ. Iowa | Comment |
|---|---|---|---|---|---|---|---|---|
| Agave found in Tex-Mex foods, tequila, margaritas, soft drinks, brown rice syrup, barley malt syrup corn syrup | | X | | X | X | X | X | |
| Any Sweetener ending in "OL" | | X | | X | | X | X | |
| Aspartame Sugar | | X | | X | X | X | X | See Notes |
| Barley Malt Syrup | X per Iowa | X | X | X | | X | X | NOTE: NOT TOLERATED IF HFI |
| Beet Sugar | | X | | X | X | X | X | |
| Brown Rice Syrup | X per Iowa | X | X | X | X | X | X | NOTE: NOT TOLERATED IF HFI |
| Brown Sugar | | X | | X | X | X | X | |
| Cane Sugar Sucrose | | X | X | X | X | X | X | NOTE: NOT TOLERATED IF HFI |
| Carmel | | X | | | | | X | |

| Food Item | Tolerated | CT= Can't Tolerate HFI individuals can't tolerate but FM may be able to tolerate | May be able to tolerate in small doses | Harvard Medical | Boston University Article/FODMAP | Mayo Clinic | Univ. Iowa | Comment |
|---|---|---|---|---|---|---|---|---|
| Confectioners' Sugar /Sucrose | | X | X Try in small dose per Iowa | X | X | X | X | A chemical combination of glucose and Fructose NOTE: NOT TOLERATED FOR HFI |
| Corn Starch | | X | | X | X | X | X | |
| Corn Syrup (Col L) | | X | | X | X | X | X | |
| Corn Syrup (Glucose Syrup) | | X | | X | X | X | X | |
| Corn Syrup Solids (Dried Glucose) | | X | | X | X | X | X | |
| Corn Syrups | | X | | X | | X | X | |
| Date Sugar | | X | | X | X | X | X | |
| Dextrin | X | | | X | X | X | X | Glucose molecules linked together in changes. Does not break down to pure dextrose |
| Dextrose | X | | | X | X | X | X | Single glucose molecule / simple sugar |

| Food Item | Tolerated | CT= Can't Tolerate HFI individuals can't tolerate but | FM may be able to tolerate May be able to tolerate in small doses | Harvard Medical | Boston University Article/FODMAP | Mayo Clinic | Univ. Iowa | Comment |
|---|---|---|---|---|---|---|---|---|
| Evaporated Cane Sugar | | X | X | X | X | X | | Sucrose made for sugar cane juice NOTE: NOT TOLERATED IF HFI |
| Fructose | | X | | X | X | X | X | Made of 6 Carbons |
| Glucose Simple Sugar | X | | | X | X | X | | Note: This is Glucose |
| Glycogen | X Per Iowa | | | | | | X | |
| Granulated Sugar | | X | X | X | X | X | | Can be tolerated if pure can sugar and not beet sugar HFI TRY WITH CAUTION |
| High Fructose Corn Syrup | | X | | X | X | X | X | |
| Honey | | X | | X | X | X | X | |
| Inverted Sugar | | X | X | | X | | X | |
| Isomalt Polyol | | X | | X | X | X | X | |
| Iszoglucose another name for HFCS | | X | | X | X | X | X | |
| Karo Syrup | | X | | | | | X | |
| Lactose | | | | | | | X | |

| Food Item | Tolerated | CT= Can't Tolerate HFI individuals can't tolerate but FM may be able to tolerate | May be able to tolerate in small doses | Harvard Medical | Boston University Article/FODMAP | Mayo Clinic | Univ. Iowa | Comment |
|---|---|---|---|---|---|---|---|---|
| Levulose | | X | | X | X | X | X | |
| Maltitol Sugar | | X | | X | X | X | X | |
| Maltose | X | | | X | X | X | X | Linked glucose molecules that rapidly break down to glucose in the intestine. |
| Maple Syrup | | X | | X | X | X | X | |
| Molasses | | X | | X | X | X | X | |
| Palm sugar | | X | | | | | X | |
| Raw Sugar | | X | X | X | X | X | | See Notes |
| Saccharin Sugar also known as Sweet n Low, Sugar Twin sucryl, Featherweight | | X | | X | X | X | X | |
| Sorbitol (Sugar Free) or "low Calorie" foods and drinks, many sweetened foods, pills and syrups check labels): maltitol or lycasin and isomalt may yield sorbitol. | | X | | X | X | X | X | |

| Food Item | Tolerated | CT= Can't Tolerate HFI individuals can't tolerate but FM may be able to tolerate | May be able to tolerate in small doses | Harvard Medical | Boston University Article/FODMAP | Mayo Clinic | Univ. Iowa | Comment |
|---|---|---|---|---|---|---|---|---|
| Splenda See Notes | | X | X | X | X | X | X | Not approved |
| Stevia See Notes | X see note | | X | X | X | X | X | No side effects, has not been tested enough at Boston University for a recommendation |
| Stevia mixed with Dextrose | X | | | | | | | Note: This is my Sweetener |
| Sucralose (Splenda) | | X | | X | X | X | X | Very Bad |
| Sucralose | | X | | X | X | X | X | Chemical name for Splenda |
| Sugar | | X | | X | | X | X | |
| Sweet Root | | X | | X | | X | X | |
| Syrups | | X | | X | | X | X | |
| Xylitol Sugar alcohol | | | X | X | X | X | X | May cause diarrhea |

Please remember everyone has their own unique body chemistry…what works for one may not work for another.

Everything on the charts has been tested using a very reliable:

## Guinea Pig…ME!

Since starting my book and testing the foods, I have found out two things to be true:

1. Fructose can still send me to the hospital
2. Doctors still need to learn about fructose

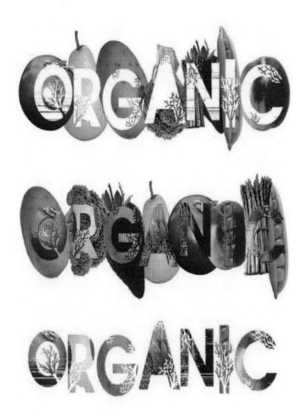

## Eat to Live!  Don't Live to Eat!

Foods with high fructose content (the examples on the next page are of some foods but not all foods). Point being made is if you look up a food item and the Glucose in the food has a higher percentage compared to the Fructose percentage…your body should be able to digest the food properly in the small intestine. When in doubt don't eat it or sample a small portion…be cautious with your selections.

Agave Syrup is Fructose

Agave syrup is pure fructose produced by industrial processing of the fructose polysaccharides in agave extracts. I cannot understand why anyone would use this commercially processed fructose as a sweetener. It doesn't raise blood sugar, because it raises blood fructose levels instead, which is much, much worse.

Aspartame Sugar: FDA approved this substitutive after an in depth study…some people experienced headaches. Current studies states this is an ingredient you don't want in your diet

Dextrin: Glucose molecules linked together in changes. Does not break down to pure dextrose, which can be processed by the small intestine.

Dextrose: Single glucose molecule / simple sugar

Evaporated Cane Sugar…may be tolerated in very small does.

Fructose: Made of 6 carbon chains

Granulated Sugar only if a 50-50 percentage ratio exists then a HFI may try with caution…must not be made of beet juice.

Iszoglucose: Another name for High Fructose Corn Syrup.

Maltose: linked glucose molecules that rapidly break down to glucose in the intestine

Raw Sugar:  Equal parts of glucose and fructose a chemical combination of glucose and fructose.  Not Tolerated if HFI

Saccharin Sugar:  Sucryl, Sweet n Low, Sugar Twin also known as Featherweight

Stevia:  Use caution the medical facilities I used for my information feel more studies must be made prior to giving this product the OK.

Sorbitol may maltitol or lycasin and isomalt may yield sorbitol

Splenda ...Boston University... hasn't been tested this enough ...at this the time of this sweetener is not considered safe.  Use caution the medical facilities I used for my information feel more studies must be made prior to giving these products the OK.

I use Stevia and it works for me.  Stevia is an herb.

Oranges:  Unclear decision from the research facilities

Raspberries and Strawberries:  Are tolerated in most people due to the Glucose/Fructose ratio, and the ability for the small intestine to breakdown this food source.

Alcohol:

If you have been diagnosed with any type of fructose issue, the following types of alcohol should be on your not tolerated list.

First thing that comes to mind is Beer!

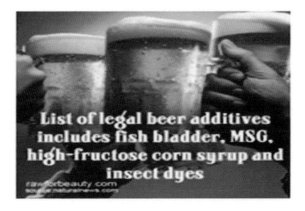

The sugar in beer is one of the worst types of sugar you can ingest. It is also a problem due to the grains used in beer because they have a high amount of fructans.

You may also want to think about this: From Raw Beauty click the link or copy, paste the link into your browser, read it, and weep. This website is everything you wanted to know about beer but was afraid to ask!

http://rawforbeauty.com/blog/list-of-legal-beer-additives-includes-fish-bladder-msg-high-fructose-corn-syrup-and-insect-dyes.html

Let me know after you read this how soon you want another beer!

Wine: Avoid any fortified wines, such as port or sherry, because of their higher fructose content.

The only wine I can drink is a dry white wine. Please note all wineries have their own "types" of dry wine so a white wine from XYZ Winery may not be suitable for you. This is a very individual need. However, if you enjoy wine please take the time to sip and see if there is a negative impact on your selection.

Hard Liquor:  Hard liquors such as vodka, rum, and whiskey do not contain fructose, unless they are flavored or sweetened. Always read the ingredient lists of any beverages, alcoholic or not, to ensure they do not contain honey or high-fructose corn syrup. You must also be careful what you mix with your liquor. Anything that is sweet or even a juice will have a very bad impact on your digestive tract.

Alcohol in general:  The general rule is the more highly refined the beverage is, the less residual sugar it will have. Stay away from cheap alcohols and fruit based brands, even if it says, "Artificially flavored" as the flavor might be artificial but the sugar content is higher to make it sweet.

Scotch whiskey, highly refined rums.   Gin can have its downfalls also.  The goal is to limit your fructose as much as possible so you can enjoy the beverage of your choice and the company of friends. Don't push your tolerance to the maximum.  If you do, you could end up damaging your digestive tract or your liver in many ways.

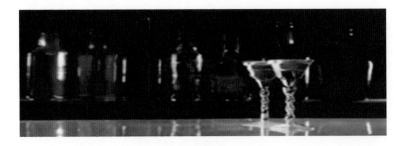

| Alcohol<br>Limit to 1 ounce for hard liquors<br>Limit to 4 ounces for Dry White Wine | Tolerated | CT= Can't Tolerate | May be able to tolerate in small doses | Harvard Medical | Boston University Sugar Reference Hereditary Fructose Intolerance | Mayo Clinic | Univ. Iowa |
|---|---|---|---|---|---|---|---|
| Gin | | | X | | | | X |
| Rum | | X | | | | | X |
| Vodka from grain or potato | | X | X | | | | X |
| Whiskey | | | X | | | | X |
| Wine Dry White | | | X | | | | X |
| Wine Red Dry | | | X | | | | X |
| Beer | | X | | | | | X |
| Wine Sweet | | X | | | | | X |

Please note: not all of the research medical facilities provided information for Alcohol.

I have researched white wines and I have found a DRY White Wine that works for me and have little if any side effects.

A protein and fat breakfast, e.g. bacon and eggs, does not produce rapid hunger, because it does not produce a large insulin rise and glucose fall. Chapter Thirteen: You Are Never "Cured"

I've included this information in my book as a "reminder" that you are never cured of your HFI or FM.

There is so much in our lives that we can't control but this…this we can control you just need to make the decision to charge of your health..

December of 2012, I was well on my way to reclaiming my life. Then I was hit with a curve ball (metaphorically speaking) I had a tooth pulled and couldn't eat anything except liquids. My problem was most liquids I couldn't digest due to fructose. Out of literal hunger, I ended up eating something that had fructose in it and I was in the hospital for the better part of 25 days.

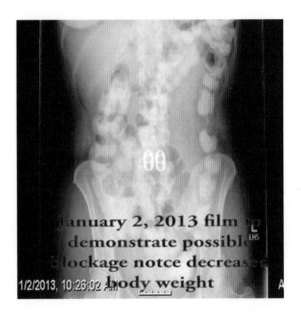

January 2, 2013 film to demonstrate possible blockage notce decrease body weight
1/2/2013, 10:26:02 AM

It was a quick and painful reminder that Hereditary Fructose Intolerance or Fructose Malabsorption is never going to be cured. I was going to have to manage this issue for the remainder of my life.

The reason for including this episode in my book was to reiterate that the medical professionals still have a long road to education and discovery regarding fructose and their treatment of patients who have this health issue.

On this bout, I was admitted 3 times in 30 days and had the misfortune of acquiring an extremely bad case of C-Diff. The C-Diff and in conjunction with my fructose problem was the cause for my multiple hospital admissions.

As I had said…I knew that I had eaten something that had fructose in it…I knew the symptoms and the horrific pain. I was rushed to the hospital. The emergency room doctors gave me nothing for pain and the hospital placed me under the care of a general surgeon. The normal tests were taken. However, no one was listening to what I had to say.

This is another strong example of what happens when the doctors don't ask how and why but instead treat the symptoms. Once again, we are simply insurance codes and numbers. Our doctor's can't take the time that they did in the past. The Insurance and Pharmaceuticals companies are calling all the shots!

The surgeon who had been appointed my case during the first and second hospital admission wanted to proceed with a surgery based on a shadow on my x-ray.

Now, in the past the shadows that the doctors thought were blockages were also considered an Ileus, a telescoping intestine…you get my point…so you can understand why I was not "Surgery" happy!

Since the onset of my HFI, I had learned that my condition could cloud the picture and perhaps even make it look like I needed surgery due the physical appearance of my intestinal tract as it looked on my x-rays. Knowing this I didn't think going blindly into the operating room was the best idea.

I told him (the Surgeon) that I wanted to look at the x-ray or scan that he based his medical decision on...he refused...telling me that I would not understand. The actual area he wanted to operate on was not that clear on the film.

His idea was to cut me from stem to stern and I quote "go through every inch of your intestines with my hands to find the problem" he abruptly left me and my husband immediately after providing us with such a wonderful picture....we sat for a moment like a deer in headlights.

My husband looked at me, broke the silence, and said to me that was never going to happen. I did two things...I prayed and called two people in the medical profession who could perhaps guide me. The next step was to fire my current surgeon. I was provided another surgeon and I explained to him that if surgery was going to take place I needed to see where the problem was on the films.

I was told surgery may still be eminent but before rushing me to surgery the new surgeon ordered a Gastrografin. This is a type of nuclear medicine where you swallow a very nasty tasting solution and then over a 5-hour period a series of x-rays are taken, each x-ray shows how the solution is travels through your small and large intestines.

The Surgeon and the technicians made sure I saw every film and I was able to watch the process of the solution going through my intestines. The result of this test was conclusive I didn't have a blockage.

What looked like an obstruction was the combination of a severe infection that had not been treated and my fructose issue.

It produced the same type of cloudiness for lack of a better word as a blockage would on a regular x-ray.

Had I been operated on with the infection...I was told it could have killed me.

You can see at the upper left side of this film that the solution I had to drink had still had not emptied out of my stomach.

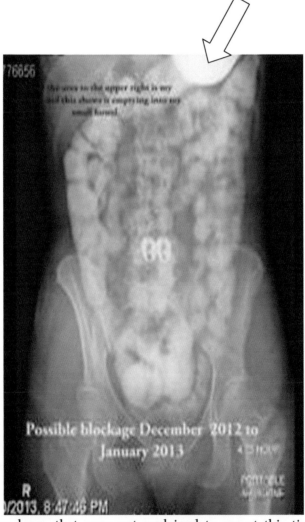

The extra loops that were not explained to me at this time were actual the cause of me having a redundant colon—this is a colon longer than most people have. I have extra loops in my large colon.

During my last admission to the hospital, a nurse who suffers from Type II diabetes asked me how I could just stop eating everything that made up my past diet.

She stated, "I could hardly stop eating just a few of the items in comparison in hopes of controlling my Type II Diabetes."

This was a good time in my life for someone to ask me that question. I provided her with a swift and simple answer…I wanted to live a full life for whatever time I may be blessed with on this earth. As they say it was a "NO Brainer"…I traded pain and the poor quality of my life for a very specific diet that would promote intestinal health.

I went on to tell the nurse that the last 20 – 25 days in and out of the hospital was an example of what happens to me if I don't stay true to my food choices.

Is the improved flavor in processed foods worth the pain? The answer was never more obvious to me than it was at that time in my life…NO!

My fructose problem is severe and the risk for me just doesn't outweigh the benefit (flavor in this case).

## A Recent Update with the Medical Community!

Approximately 20 months later and I find that Doctors, Nurses, and Hospitals still have a great deal to learn when it comes to Fructose and the pain associated with this illness.

As I continue to create recipes for my own use, I find that being the "Guinea Pig" has its ups and its downs.

Twice during the last 8 months, I have ingested fructose in the line of creating my recipes and it has placed me in the ER. The ER staff is still not listening to what is being said to them.

I tell them what is wrong, they look at me like deer in headlights, and once I get that reaction I know I am dealing with someone who doesn't have a clue!

The last time I was in the Emergency Room I took a rough draft of my book and gave it to the ER Doctor.

I told the ER staff what was wrong, what I needed, and why I need it. I told them I could not take any form of codeine and that certain antispasmodic medication (Bentyl in my case) could not be tolerated. I even told them why I could not tolerate the medication.

The response I received from the medical professionals on both occasions was one of extreme irritation and resentment.

How could I as a patient tell them the "Professionals" what to do?

From a personal standpoint I can say I know more about my Digestive Tract than someone who has never seen me before or someone who is simply looking at my history.

They never experienced the 2 ½ years of hell and I will continue to stand my ground.

When they released me, I was sent home with Bentyl and hydro-codeine! Neither medication is tolerated in my system. I explained this upfront and it was totally ignored.

Education within the Medical Community is paramount!

I continue to read and research issues regarding our foods and hidden dangers of our modern technology in the kitchen. My book would not be complete unless I mentioned a few additional issues. There are "other" dangers to our current food selections. It is important to share how relevant those dangers are to our health.

Once I created my Fructose-Specific Food Charts, I knew I only had one direction and that was forward. I no longer deal with all of the confusion and whiplash from the multiple diagnoses. I found my voice and I stopped Kvetching and took action! I was in control of my life! This is what I want for you!

I can guarantee you that your energy and mental health will vastly improve with these changes. There is no magic pill for improving your health...you must make these choices on your own. I enjoy everything I CAN EAT!

## Start Feeling Better Now!

I suggest that you ask your doctor to do a blood panel on you to see what you may need in your diet to make the most of what you eat. If you're deficient in any vitamins or minerals, you need to know that up front.

Make sure every meal counts. Include protein in all of your meals. Empty calories are something you don't need.

I mentioned this briefly before. A strategy for selecting positive food choices i.e. choosing foods in which fructose and glucose are in balance OR have more glucose than fructose.

Co-ingestion strategies included co-ingestion of free glucose to balance excess free fructose problematic foods.

Co-ingestions of alanine-rich foods (**) was not a standard practice because it was considered a more difficult concept for patients to understand and implement and it was less practical.

I don't agree with this statement because I believe educating the patient will allow them to better understand how their body works...don't allow anyone to short change your level of intelligence.

Note: alanine, in its essence, is a form of amino acid that is found in protein-rich foods, mainly in foods such as pork, beef, and other meats. While it is often found in protein-rich foods, it is not a protein-building amino acid in and of itself. However, increasing the amount of beta alanine in your blood stream can also raise the level of carnosine in your blood, and carnosine is the active agent in the body that can help to build lean muscle mass and improve athletic endurance and performance. Carnosine acts as a tissue and cellular buffer during workouts and helps to block the effects of increased lactic acid production that can cause muscle fatigue. (33)

Question how your food is manufactured and/or preserved the process can negatively affect your health.

You may want to consider using a nutritionist. Since a nutritionist is, a person who studies how food works in the body...this would be a great match for someone who is educated in regards to their food choices but may not feel comfortable with doing it on their own.

A nutritionist study how nutritional deficiencies cause and support illness and how to turn it around with a "let food be the medicine" approach as taught by Hippocrates, the ancient Greek physician known as the father of medicine.

Making this type of lifestyle change is compared to trying to swim upstream and some may find it impossible to do on their own.

We have been trained to eat fast, chemically infused food which is now part of our culture and will continue to beckon you... junk food have been made part of our social life "eat whatever is the fastest and most convenient" regardless of the health issues...we want something that will fit into our hectic lives.

We have lost touch with what real foods from the earth can contribute because chemicals in the foods we have been eating for years have hijacked our brains. We all need to re-train our brains to eat healthy!

I have removed GMO's and Trans fats from my diet.

A recent survey shows that more than 190 million adult Americans are incorporating low calorie foods and sugar-free foods and beverages into their meal plan as what they think is a healthier lifestyle change. The truth these are not healthy lifestyle changes the sugar-free low or zero fat and unnecessary additives in our foods are making us sick and fat.

I understand if you have IBS or other digestive issues how frustrating it can be to follow a diet due to the lack of valid information. They even provide conflicting information…they keep you confused intentionally. Who is "they"…they be the advertising companies!

Truth in Advertising – you can't always believe what you see in advertising…they make a convincing case but in regards to our food we, the consumer get the short end of the stick!

## Sugar Makes You Hungry

The human body can only use simple sugars, e.g. glucose, fructose, sucrose, or starch.

Body enzymes convert sucrose into fructose + glucose, and starch into glucose. Other carbs, such as soluble fiber, are only digested by gut bacteria in the colon.

The conversion of starches to glucose begins with enzymes in saliva in the mouth and is completed in the upper part of the digestive tract. Starch should be considered as a simple sugar, because it causes a rapid rise in blood sugar, just like glucose. It may actually be faster than table sugar.

The rapid rise of blood sugar causes a rapid increase in blood insulin, which in turn rapidly removes sugar into fat cells. The rapid rise and fall of blood sugar provides the experience of hunger.

That is why cereal, e.g. at meal, in the morning produces intense hunger just a few hours later. Actually, oatmeal is a bit healthier than most cereals, because it also has some sol

*We all crave sugar but do you understand why we crave sugar?*

Sugar enters the bloodstream and stimulates the same pleasure centers of the brain hat respond to heroin and cocaine.

All sweet yummy types of food do this to an extent…that is why it is so appetizing. However, sugar has acute shocking effect. Some have written that sugar is literally is an addictive drug.

Over thousands of years, our bodies have gone through a type of mutation that has evolved into a will-oiled machine we have today.

Sugar is like sex…once you tried and you like it…you want more and more you have the more you want!

Our bodies have always needed a small amount of fructose. Our bodies have reached the point that we need very little fructose because how extremely efficient our bodies are in processing a natural amount of fructose. Therefore, a small amount goes along way.

Fructose issues can't be fixed with pharmaceuticals or modern medicine as we think of it today.

It is up to YOU to control your eating habits and that is plain common sense…do you want to spend thousands of dollars of medication or eat healthy?

*It is simple…either spend your money on prescriptions or on food…I choose food!*

219

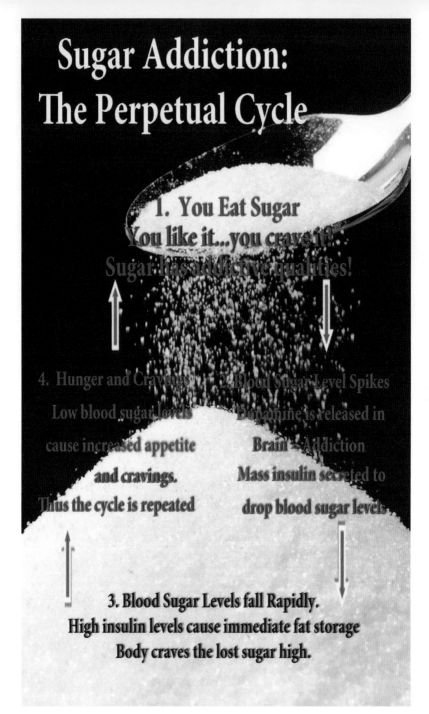

# Sugar Addiction:
# The Perpetual Cycle

**1. You Eat Sugar**
You like it...you crave it!
Sugar has addictive qualities!

**4. Hunger and Cravings**
Low blood sugar levels
cause increased appetite
and cravings.
Thus the cycle is repeated

**2. Blood Sugar Level Spikes**
Dopamine is released in
Brain = Addiction
Mass insulin secreted to
drop blood sugar levels

**3. Blood Sugar Levels fall Rapidly.**
High insulin levels cause immediate fat storage
Body craves the lost sugar high.

IBS, Extreme Fatigue, Autism, Alzheimer's Disease

GERD/Acid Reflux, Irritable Bowel Syndrome, FODMAPS, Gastritis Support, Obesity, Type II Diabetes, Hereditary Fructose Intolerance, Candida, Leaky Gut, Depression, Chronic Inflammation, Gluten, and Celiac, and The Brain-Gut Connection

I'm more alarmed than ever about the dangers of high fructose corn syrup. This cheap sugar alternative, which is made from cornstarch, is seriously bad news. It's another fabricated toxic burden for the body, and probably worse for our health than we ever thought.

HFCS serves not only as a sugar alternative, but also as a means to enhance a product's shelf life. As such, food manufacturers use it in practically everything. Soft drinks and processed foods are especially notorious for it, as are canned foods (even, as it turns out, my precious canned beans). On average, Americans consume about 12 teaspoons of HFCS per day, or approximately 1 in every 10 calories.

The list of potential dangers of high fructose corn syrup is long. The more you consume, the more you put your liver, kidneys and arteries at risk; the more likely you are to put on weight; and the more prone you become to metabolic syndrome, a forerunner to diabetes, hypertension, autoimmune illnesses, and heart disease.

When I discovered HFCS was in my canned goods...all canned goods were discarded!

I had just read that the environmental medicine conference in Dallas had a speaker named Jean Monro, M.D., a British physician who had spoken about HFCS. She reported that about 25 percent of her patients with metabolic syndrome lack enough of the enzymes needed to process HFCS, either because of a genetic defect, or because they'd consumed so much of the substance that their enzymes had become exhausted and ineffective.

The inability to properly process HFCS often leads to an increase in the level of uric acid in the body. Uric acid is a normal product of cellular breakdown, but too much of it can lead to health problems. Most significantly, it can inhibit the ability of endothelial cells to produce nitric oxide—a substance that's crucial for keeping arteries properly dilated. In fact, the connection between fructose and uric acid is regarded as a potential cause of high blood pressure and kidney disease (a common side effect of chronic hypertension). The link has also been reported in medical literature in relation to fructose-induced metabolic syndrome.

The first place to look is in the gut because 75 percent of the body's immune system activity comes from the gut.

At the Arizona Center for Advanced Medicine, they identify foods and other substances (chemicals, pollens, molds) which cause gut inflammation in the individual, and work to eliminate the responsible foods from the patient's environment. They look at the body burden of heavy metals like mercury, arsenic and lead, and make every effort to eliminate these as well, since they can be a significant cause of inflammatory response. They can provide supplements and remedies to correct the dysfunctional information systems in the body, and to heal the GI tract and improve its overall health. They show you how colonics and probiotics (note: Some probiotics have fructose as an ingredient) work to replace the damaging bacteria in the gut with ones, which are actively helpful. Finally, they look at brain function, to help modify the effect of the autonomic nervous system (the stress system) on the gut. Thus, the GI tract is restored, symptoms are cleared, and health returns.

Most Americans today have weakened and impaired immune systems that are unable to function as they were designed. Experts estimate that many allergies and immune-system diseases have doubled, tripled or even quadrupled in the last few decades. Some studies indicate that more than half of the U.S. population has at least one allergy.

Asthma, hay fever, eczema and food allergies are all "allergic diseases" caused by your immune system responding to substances that are ordinarily harmless, such as pollen or peanuts. Autoimmune diseases also result from your body's defense mechanisms malfunctioning, causing your immune system to attack parts of your body such as your nerves, pancreas or digestive tract.

Some researchers suspect the rise in immune system dysfunctions may have a common explanation rooted in aspects of modern living. The first item mentioned is High Fructose Corn Syrup.

First, we have undergone a revolutionary change in how we fuel our body. For tens of thousands of years, mankind ate unprocessed, truly natural food. In the last 150 years or so, our diets have changed dramatically. Our genes simply cannot adapt that quickly. The human body is not designed to run on 150 pounds per year of processed sugar, nor is it designed to run on baby formula, aspartame, pesticides, hydrogenated oils or meat from animals fed unnatural diets and hormones. Sugar for example, impairs the intestinal micro flora and undermines a strong immune system.

## II. DIFFERENT WAYS IMMUNE SYSTEM DYSFUNCTION SHOWS UP

- Arthritis
- Leaky gut
- Multiple Sclerosis
- Lupus
- Chronic fatigue syndrome
- Inflammatory bowel disease (Crohn's and Ulcerative Colitis)
- Scleroderma

- Osteoarthritis is characterized by destruction of cartilage within the joint, eventually exposing the underlying bone. The cells, which produce cartilage for unknown reasons, fail to maintain the balance between production and destruction of normal cartilage tissue. Compounds called proteoglycans form the cartilage itself, and these proteins are found to be deficient in cartilage from patients with osteoarthritis. Other compounds called metalloproteinases are also found in high concentration in osteoarthritic cartilage. These compounds digest proteoglycans. Metallothioneins are proteins normally present all over the body. Their functions include storing high concentrations of zinc, scavenging free radicals, protecting against cadmium toxicity. These proteins are known to be neuroprotective, probably through their ability to scavenge free radicals.

- Rheumatoid arthritis for most patients is a progressive disability. RA is associated with several genes, the most familiar of which is the HLA gene. It appears to be influenced by multiple factors, including diet, inflammation, bacterial infection, and heavy metals. Standard allopathic treatment involves use of steroids and sometimes anti-neoplastic drugs. If anti-inflammatory therapy is initiated before joint deformities are present, it is possible to avoid the joint deformities entirely. Some patients treated with antibiotics for months have improved their arthritis symptoms. However, the use of long term steroids and other anti-inflammatories have led to suppressed immune system, candida overgrowth, peptic ulcers and other problems. Determination of food sensitivities and heavy metal toxicities is crucial. For many, remission has not been possible without dietary changes, particularly elimination of sugar and grains. Additionally, chronic mycoplasma infections must be investigated.

- Spondyloarthropathies (ankylosing spondylitis is the best known of this group) involve primarily the vertebrae and the joints between the sacrum and the pelvis below the low back (SI joint). There is peripheral joint inflammation, mainly of the larger joints (knees or hips), rather than the smaller joints (hands) as typically seen in osteoarthritis. This form of arthritis is frequently associated with inflammatory bowel disease, inflammation of the eye (uveitis), and skin diseases like psoriasis. Genetics is thought to play a significant role in this form of arthritis. HLA B27 is found in 90% of patients with ankylosing spondylitis.

A clear association has been found in some patients between arthritis and inflammatory bowel disease. Patients with increased intestinal permeability ("leaky gut") have a higher incidence of arthritis. If you have abused our colons for years through an unhealthy diet, or if we have developed food sensitivities, constipation and colitis, it only makes sense to treat the colon to improve the Leaky gut.

Most Americans today have weakened and impaired immune systems that are unable to function as they were designed. Experts estimate that many allergies and immune-system diseases have doubled, tripled or even quadrupled in the last few decades. Some studies indicate that more than half of the U.S. population has at least one allergy.

Asthma, hay fever, eczema and food allergies are all "allergic diseases" caused by your immune system responding to substances that are ordinarily harmless, such as pollen or peanuts. Autoimmune diseases also result from your body's defense mechanisms malfunctioning, causing your immune system to attack parts of your body such as your nerves, pancreas or digestive tract. ( (35)

This chapter will explain GMO's, problems with our Labeling system in our country and provide to you some miscellaneous items that didn't seem to fit anywhere else!

As I have explained in previous chapter fructose, affects everyone on some level. From Fructose Malabsorption, Digestive Tract, Heart, Brain, Autism, Alzheimer's, ADD and ADHD and the list goes on.

I have all ready tied additional health issues in with Fructose due to the huge impact Fructose has on everyone and the ability that Fructose has to mimic other health issues in our system. One final topic is Genetically Modified Organisms.

### What is a GMO and How Does it Affect Us?

A genetically modified organism (GMO) is an organism whose genetic material has been altered using genetic engineering techniques. Organisms that have been genetically modified include microorganisms such as bacteria and yeast, insects, plants, fish, and Mammals.

GMOs are genetically modified foods, and are widely used in scientific research, as well as, to produce goods other than food.

The term GMO is very close to the technical legal term, 'living modified organism' defined in the Cartagena Protocol on Bio-safety, which regulates international trade in living GMOs (specifically, "any living organism that possesses a novel combination of genetic material obtained through the use of modern biotechnology")

*This too affects our digestive system in many similar ways!*

Genetic engineering focuses on the history and methods of genetic engineering, and on applications of genetic engineering and of GMOs. There are separate articles on genetically modified crops, genetically modified food, regulation of the release of genetic modified organisms, and controversies.

Genetic modification involves the mutation, insertion, or deletion of genes. When genes are inserted, they usually come from a different species, which is a form of horizontal gene transfer.

In nature, this can occur when exogenous DNA penetrates the cell membrane for any reason. Intended host with a very small syringe, or with very small particles fired from a gene gun. However, other methods exploit natural forms of gene.

To do this artificially may require attaching the genes to a virus or just physically inserting the extra DNA into the nucleus of the transfer, such as the ability of Agro bacterium to transfer genetic material to plants or the ability of lentiviruses to transfer genes to animal cells.

Uses

GMOs are used in biological and medical research, production of pharmaceutical drugs, experimental medicine (e.g. gene therapy), and agriculture (e.g. golden rice, resistance to herbicides). The term "genetically modified organism" does not always imply, but can include, targeted insertions of genes from one species into another.

Such methods are useful tools for biologists in many areas of research, including those who study the mechanisms of human and other diseases or fundamental biological processes in eucaryotic or prokaryotic cells.

In agriculture, genetically engineered crops are created to possess several desirable traits, such as resistance to pests, herbicides, or harsh environmental conditions, improved product shelf life, increased nutritional value, or production of valuable goods such as drugs (pharming).

Since the first commercial cultivation of genetically modified plants in 1996, they have been modified to be tolerant to the herbicides glufosinate and glyphosate, to be resistant to virus damage as in Ringspot virus-resistant GM papaya, grown in Hawaii, and to produce the BT toxin, an insecticide that is documented as non-toxic to mammals.

Critics have objected to GM crops per se on several grounds, including ecological concerns, and economic concerns raised by the fact these organisms are subject to intellectual property law.

GM crops also are involved in controversies over GM food with respect to whether food produced from GM crops is safe and whether GM crops are needed to address the world's food needs.

The genetically modified foods controversy is a dispute over the relative advantages and disadvantages of food derived from genetically modified organisms, genetically modified crops used to produce food and other goods, and other uses of genetically modified organisms in food production.

The dispute involves consumers, biotechnology companies, governmental regulators, non-governmental organizations, and scientists.

The key areas of controversy related to genetically modified (GM) food is the risk of harm to people and animals that ingest these products. Moreover, should GM foods be labeled?

The role of government regulators are to monitor the effect of levels GM crops on the environment, the effect on pesticide resistance, the impact of GM crops for farmers, including farmers in developing countries, the role of GM crops in feeding the growing world population, and GM crops as part of the industrial agriculture system.

If it is a genetically modified organism, the DNA has changed and that food now has a different effect on your body and digestive system.

This is a fact. That is why so many people are going organic. For an example look at the chicken in your grocery store...if the chicken breasts are huge...they have been feed GMO grains.

Look at the organic chicken breasts...they are much smaller but that is the way chicken looked 30 years ago. If a manufactured molecule made that chicken breast so much larger what do, you think it is doing to your intestinal tract and your body in general.

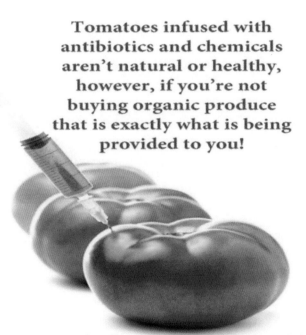

**Tomatoes infused with antibiotics and chemicals aren't natural or healthy, however, if you're not buying organic produce that is exactly what is being provided to you!**

**Eat Fresh, Organic & Healthy Foods!**

Genetically modified organisms also known as (GMO's) can be found in as many as 60-70% of the foods in the US.

As we have written about in the past dangers of GMO's, a genetically modified organism according to The Non-GMO Project are organisms that have been created through the gene-splicing techniques of biotechnology (also called genetic engineering or GE.

This relatively new science allows DNA from one species to be injected into another species in a lab, creating combination's of plant, animal, bacteria, and viral genes that do not occur in nature or through traditional crossbreeding methods. The use of genetically modified organisms in foods was recently banned in Europe, but the US isn't to that point yet due to the highly political nature of what is keeping GMO's on the market and in our food.

Here are six of the dangers that have been discovered by consuming genetically modified foods

1. Food Allergy Symptoms Increase Dramatically

According to scientific research, it has been shown that those who eat genetically modified foods tend to see an increase in their allergic reactions to the types of foods they are already allergic too. By eating these genetically modified foods people also form allergies to foods which they

2. Bodily Toxicity Increases

As individuals ingest more and more genetically modified foods and organisms into their body it has been shown that the bodies toxicity increases which leads to a ton of other potentially serious health problems. As stated by NaturalNews.com it has been shown that there is a definite link between Obesity, Cancer, and Toxicity.

### 3. Negative Reproductive Effects

In lab tests done on animals there were cases where once the animals ingested genetically modified food they became completely sterile in a matter of weeks. What was interesting in fact was that in some cases these animals were force fed the food because they didn't want to eat it themselves naturally.

### 4. Negative Effect to Digestive System

They are finding that GMO's are a breeding ground for bacteria and viruses and since the digestive system is where the body is exposed when ingesting these harmful foods, reversing the damaging effects of these foods is nearly impossible.

In other cases on mice and rats, there is documented proof that the digestive system grows bigger for some strange reason. I could relate to this comment and I'm human.

### 5. Unknown Genetic Effects on Humans

The jury is still out on all of the known causes about how Genetically Modified Organisms will negatively affect the greater human race, so it would be best to avoid them at all costs knowing the long-term health risks of ingesting these foods on a regular basis.

6. Death…In some cases death has also been a challenge in working with GMO foods where rats and mice die in a matter of weeks by eating genetically modified food.

As everything adds up over time, and the more these genetically modified foods are pushed on us as Americans, knowing the dangers going in and actively speaking out against it may save more lives now and in the future.

You care about your health, and you're vigilant of the fact that foods that have been genetically modified have been shown to <u>cause allergies, organ failure, and general toxicity</u>. Therefore, it should be essential such scary flippen-foods be avoided. To not only better your own health but also <u>prevent mineral-loss in soil</u> from conventional growing methods, take care to buy the following foods organic, or avoid them altogether.

1. Soy:  Many food options are supplemented with soy, but it is one of the most common foods to be grown genetically modified. (<u>Current statistics</u> state 93% of soy in the US is modified). Look at the ingredient list...if your non-organic product contains soy flour, lecithin, or soy protein isolate and concentrates (protein shakes), it's likely been obtained from a GMO source. Many products also contain soy derivatives: Vitamin E supplements, tofu, cereals, veggie burgers, soy sausages, tamari, soy sauce, chips, ice cream, frozen yogurt, protein powder, margarine, soy cheese, crackers, breads, cookies, chocolates, candy, fried foods, shampoo, cosmetics, enriched flours, pastas, and even bubble bath. Its use in so many products is concerning, so be sure to choose food products grown as sustainably as possible if you choose to include it in your diet.

2. Corn:  This staple may be the number one crop grown in the US, but nearly <u>88 percent</u> of what's harvested is genetically modified. It's commonly found in products that utilize corn flour, cornstarch, corn oil, corn sweeteners, and syrups.  Some examples of such foods are Vitamin C supplements, corn chips, candy, ice cream, infant formula, salad dressings, tomato sauces, bread, cookies, cereals, baking powder, alcohol, vanilla, margarine, soy sauce, soda, fried foods, powdered sugar, enriched flours, and pastas.

It's quite clear: buy (or grow!) organic corn, or leave it out of your diet.

3. Cotton:   Cotton is a crop that is commonly grown genetically modified. Its use is mainly for oil and fabrics, but such products that may contain genetically modified derivatives include: clothes, liners, chips, peanut butter, crackers, and cookies.

4. Canola:   This food source is mainly utilized for oil. However, products that may contain GMO derivatives include a wide variety of what you might buy at the supermarket: processed foods, chips, crackers, cereal, snack bars, frozen foods, canned soups, candy, breads, hummus, and some oil blends.

Great alternative options for baking or cooking are coconut and/or olive oil, which have lower cooking heat temperatures (lower heat temperature means high-heated foods can become carcinogenic) but boast many health benefits.

5. Sugar Beets:   These sweet beets are utilized for their sugar, but can cause nasty side effects if grown GMO. If any product does not specify "cane sugar" on their ingredient list, chances are you are obtaining sugar from sweets beets.   The reason sugar from beets is harmful is due to the fact the sugar is extracted from the beet and removing the natural fiber which in turn makes this type of sugar hard for you liver to digest.

Example products include cookies, cakes, ice cream, donuts, baking mixes, candy, juice, and yogurt.

6. Alfalfa:   This green crop is the fourth largest to be grown in the US, but very often is genetically modified. While grown mainly to feed to cattle (therefore in all conventionally raised meat), it's also common in pork, poultry, eggs, and dairy.

7. Aspartame:   This dangerous artificial sweetener should be avoided at all costs.

Not only has it been shown to decrease the immune system and contribute to <u>behavioral disorders</u> in children, it's genetically modified. Such sources it's found in include diet soda soft drinks, diet foods, and yogurt.

8. Dairy:   Cows raised for milking in conventional farms are commonly treated with the growth hormone RBGH. While its effect on humans is still being argued, it's been clearly shown that it has a negative effect on the cows that have been injected with it.

You can find this questionable additive in all conventionally raised dairy products: milk, cheese, yogurt, butter, ice cream, and whey.

9. Papaya:   While sweet and filling, <u>75% of the Hawaiian papaya crop</u> is genetically modified to withstand the papaya Ringspot virus. Because of this, it's not recommended to consume the fruit unless it's been sourced organically.

To prevent common health illnesses, which are completely avoidable through <u>dietary change and lifestyle choices</u>, choose foods that are unprocessed, organically produced, and if possible, locally sourced. Once again, if you have a Whole Foods this will meet and exceed your requirements.

Avoiding the commonly genetically modified foods will serve you and your family's health best in the present and future.

Remember, you can only be sure you are eating the above items completely GMO-free by purchasing them from farms certified-Organic, growing them yourself, or by attaining them from establishments verified by the <u>Non-GMO Project</u>.

In the end, you have to make your own decision!

If a food source is chemically altered and the DNA has been affected, it doesn't belong in your system. Your system will not process it and if your body does not process the food source properly, it will be stored as fat and create health issues in many areas. I have stated this often and in many ways but unless your life is hanging in "limbo," many will not take heed to this advice.

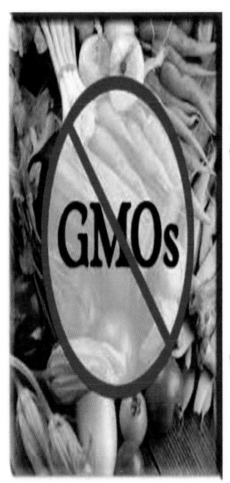

Discover the real difference between organic foods and their traditionally grown counter parts when it comes to nutrition, safety and your overall health!
This is not a fad...eating fresh organic food is healthier for anyone. We need to control and reduce the amount of chemicals that we put in our bodies...your life could depend on it!

Eat Organic and help heal yourself.

Advertising, Food Conglomerates, Pharmaceuticals, Medical Profession

For as long as anyone can remember the "advertising world" has told us how to feel, look, dress, eat, smoke, drink and what medications we should take. We enjoyed the aesthetically pleasing ads and commercials and whether you were consciously aware of "it" you were being programmed to think what "they" wanted you to think based on who had the deepest pockets in corporate America.

This has not changed but the message that is provided to "us" the consumer needs to be honest when it comes to our *health*. We unfortunately always seem to take the bait, hook, line and sinker and at some point, we need precise answers to some very basic questions. Are certain products negatively affecting our health? I don't want the advertising companies to think for me or direct me to something that will hurt my health or that of my family based on a message from the Food Conglomerates they work for…I want a message that forces someone…if they are wrong…to take responsibility. Currently, that is not happening.

"We" as a whole have gotten complacent when it comes to how we treat our bodies. We want to eat and drink to excess and have a "magic" pill to take the next day to "fix" what we allowed to take place. The majority of us went down the primrose path willingly and we must shoulder the responsibility of the current state of our health.

Welcome to the world of pharmaceuticals! Did we not see this coming? Were we so happy to be able to openly graze on whatever we wanted and really think there was no consequence at the end of the day?

The pharmaceuticals and I dare same many physicians at some point decided it was more profitable to give the public a pill for their unbridled appetite then it was to simply tell people…that it(it being a food selection) is not good for you and you are sick because you could not make the correct decision. Hell, how can you make money from that thought process?

Therefore, ranging from the medical profession, pharmaceutical companies, the food conglomerates, and the sake of the Holy ever-lasting bottom line…we collectively have been brought to a health crisis in this country. The food conglomerates provided us with zero-calorie and fat-free product…did it occur to many of us just what in the hell did we think we were eating? If it doesn't have real food that has fat and sugar, it has chemicals that have replaced those ingredients and the majority of us never questioned that…we were just happy to see that someone provided us with a way that we could just eat all we wanted. At some point, the piper must be paid and the piper is here to collect.

We have health issues that have far surpassed the projected numbers from 30 years ago. We see a rise in many illnesses that go hand and hand with the chemically laded food in our processed world. As the consumption of processed/chemical laded foods, increase so to the health issues. Why does that seem to be a flawed thought process? Why do people think that this is such a far- fetched idea?

The medical profession knew their patients were developing health issues and then… as our saving grace…in jumped the pharmaceutical companies to provide a quick fix for our problems, but at what cost?

You can't turn on your Flat Screen, Internet, Facebook, or any other device without seeing a "new" medication for your current ailment.

Moreover, for those of you who haven't noticed we have new aliments all the time. Do you ever listen to the list of side effects that are quickly rolled out with each Ad? If each prescription has an average of a dozen side effects and if you are, taking on an average 4 meds a month then it is possible that out of the possible 48 side effects…does it not occur to you that you could possibly be creating havoc on your body.

At what point do we take responsibility for our actions and say enough is enough?

The current debate about sugar, fat, High Fructose Corn Syrup and Genetically Modified Food should be rather simple. If the research was done to provide us with a truthful answer and performed solely by medical researchers who's intention was to get to the bottom of these debates and provide us with a "real" answer…that would clear up the constant confusion and wavering of what is the truth. We need "Medical Science not Medical Industry" providing us with the research. Trust me there is a huge difference.

Unfortunately, many of the studies are paid for by the companies that produce the food that happens to be the very food in question. I don't believe for one minute you will get an honest response when their bottom line is at stake. Any report can be skewed to support an argument especially with the kind of money that is at stake!

And if you think there isn't mass confusion go on line to one of many sites regarding multiple health issues you will see such mass confusion that it will make your head spin. One on-line site will tell an item is OK to eat and the next list states that it isn't…so how do you know what is right. My method to cut to the chase was to ask two questions…did a company own the site. Was a product being sold on the site? If I found that to be the case, I quickly left the group.

I found if you posted something on a company or product based site that the administrator of that site jumped on you telling you that there was only one way to think and that was their way…not for me. I think the need to remember the little thing called "Freedom of Speech.

The Advertising, Pharmaceutical, Food Conglomerates must be laughing at how they have us chasing our tails. I am the first to admit that for every piece of research I found that was against High Fructose Corn Syrup and Genetically Modified Foods…someone else could provide me with a list that countered the prior information I had found.

One thing that jumped out at me was the following; all the research that has been done from the prominent research facilities could provide me with concrete information that fit the explosion of health issues that went hand and hand with increased consumption of HFCS and GMO's. Therefore, that made sense to me regarding what I was reading and supported that side of the argument. However, for every article that argued on behalf of HFCS and GMO's—clearly stating that "their" research proved that there wasn't a connection between the consumption of these items and the increase of the health issues—not once could that research explain why we are seeing such an avalanche of these health issues.

We are seeing a tremendous rise in Digestive Disorders, Depression, Obesity, Childhood Obesity, Type II Diabetes, Autism, Alzheimer's disease and other health issues and the only commonality is they have risen in conjunction with the increased consumption of HFCS and GMO's. If someone on the side of this issue, who supports the use of these products can explain to me, as well as, thousands of others that this is merely a coincidence then I am all ears.

I am guilty of what I said in the Forward of my book... People will never truly understand something until it happens to them!

## A Flaw in Our Thought Process?

I have noticed some very flawed thinking when it comes to rationalizing our health issues. People think if there is a pill or surgery to fix it (it being whatever the health concern may be) why not just going on making poor judgment calls. I spoke to more than a dozen people who had heart by-pass surgery to save their lives. The comments that came out of their mouths were astounding. Quote, "Now, that I'm fixed and they have new medication I can eat whatever I want!" Amazingly flawed and unfortunately shared by many—this was the response from many!

Unfortunately, that is how many of us think...lets ruin our health today because I can take a pill tomorrow!

I have research from Harvard, Boston University, Sloan Kettering, University of Iowa, Mayo Clinic, Cleveland Clinic, University of Southern California, Oxford and additional research from Canada and England...that have provided me with an answer. Simply put it "Cause & Effect." If you are eating, processed foods then switch to eating organic natural foods you feel better. I have not found one person who can argue that point.

Thousands of people have digestive disorders that can't be explained by the Medical Community other than...Irritable Bowel Syndrome...hell yes my Bowel is irritable I have been placing chemicals into my system that can't be processed the way our body was meant to process food. Therefore, our bodies are confused and overloaded with toxins and the result is a nation on the brink of a catastrophic health decline.

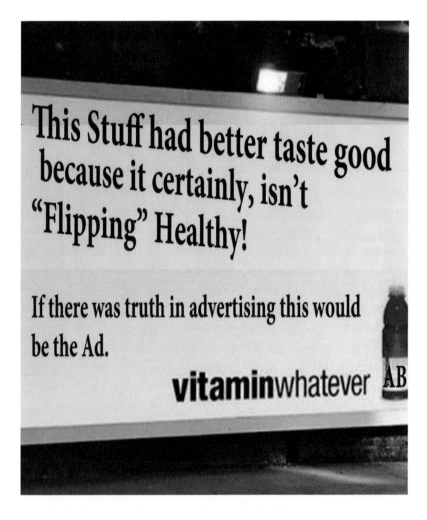

Producers of processed food in most countries, including the USA, are not currently required by law to mark foods containing "fructose in excess of glucose." This can cause some surprises and pitfalls for fructose Malabsorbers.

Genetically engineered food genes transferring to our own genes could lead to many health issues...because GM foods are not required to be labeled as such, it's impossible for consumers to tell them apart from regular foods.

Currently, there is a movement to petition the FDA, FDA to give consumers a choice. More than 600,000 people have already signed.

Current Example from Recent Headlines:

As of Today: Washington State Vote to Label GM Food Defeated by Corporations "Sophisticated Propaganda Machine

Monday, 11 November 2013 10:42 by Juan Gonzalez and Amy Goodman, Democracy Now! | Video Report: The campaign against Initiative 522 drew millions of dollars from major corporations and out-of-state organizations that spent more than $22 million to defeat it, including Monsanto, which donated more than $5 million, and DuPont, which gave almost $4 million. Pepsi, Coca-Cola, and Nestle dedicated more than $1.5 million each. This comes as a recent New York Times poll found 93 percent of Americans want labels on food containing GM ingredients. Sixty-four countries require it.

In between cells, are desmosomes, which keep the cells together, forming a strong structure preventing large molecules from passing through? When an area becomes inflamed, the structure is weakened, allowing larger molecules to escape. The makes the immune system produce antibodies and cytokines to fight off molecules because they are perceived as antigens.

Allergies have already skyrocketed in the US, and with the introduction of GE soy in the UK, soy related allergies rose to 50%. Yet federal agencies ignore the dangers of genetic engineering. See more at http://www.anh-usa.org/genetically-engineered-food-alters-our-digestive-systems/#sthash.33VVSMXg.dpuf

# What will it take for you to eat healthy?

Nancie Paruso Hyper-sensitive Theory

## Thought Process

Either we never heard of many of our Autoimmune Diseases, and Food Intolerances thirty years ago or the percentage of individuals in 1970 was so small it wasn't mentioned much by the medical community.

The individuals who now comprise hundreds of thousands of individuals afflicted by the various health issues have skyrocketed past the projected numbers provided by actuaries years ago.

## Theory

I have a theory regarding the rise of most of the Digestive Diseases, as well as, the increase in Obesity, Type II Diabetes, Autism, Autoimmune Diseases and even Alzheimer's.

I believe the change in our diets over the last 30+ years with the introduction of High Fructose Corn Syrup, GMO's, and Inulin into all of our processed food—which includes all "Fast Food" has left our bodies in a hyper-sensitive state, as well as, a chronic state of inflammation opening the door for the avalanche of sick people in our country. I personally feel that it is irrefutable that the food additives are the culprit to the current state of health in our country.

Some researchers suspect the rise in immune system dysfunctions may have a common explanation rooted in aspects of modern living. The first item I mention is High Fructose Corn Syrup.

First, we have undergone a revolutionary change in how we fuel our body. Our bodies are designed to burn fructose very efficiently. It is a process that for tens of thousands of years, mankind ate unprocessed, truly natural food. In the last 40 years or so, our diets have changed dramatically.

Our genes simply cannot adapt that quickly. The human body is not designed to run on 150 pounds per year of processed sugar, nor is it designed to run on sugar supplements like, aspartame, pesticides, hydrogenated oils or meat from animals fed unnatural diets and hormones.

Our diets are so nutritionally bad for us—by eating all of the chemically laded food; we have made our body's hyper-sensitive to even natural elements in our diet. Our bodies are in a constant state of inflammation, which accounts for the poor health this country is dealing with.

This how I feel we reached this point in our health.

## HFCS, GMO's, Synthetic Inulin, Overload of Sugar

### Sweeteners

We were ecstatic that we had sweeteners that had no calories…we didn't stop to think what those calories were being replaced with. Why would we…we just got a free pass to drink or eat whatever we wanted with no added calories…we were in nirvana!

Once the Food Conglomerates and Advertising sunk their teeth in to this untapped market, it was pure gold,

Suddenly, everything seemed to provide us with the "zero" calorie selection. You were given the choice of sugar or zero calories…of course we all jumped on the zero calories.

### Fat Free

Once again, the Food Conglomerates found a substitute for "FAT!" Now they could sell fat-free, sugar free—literally calorie free food. Once again, no one was asking what the substitution was for us to enjoy something we normally would not pig out on and it was more CHEMICALS!

## Fiber/Inulin

Ah—fiber...it was yet another loss for good nutrition.

I started seeing products that were now better for you because they had Fiber added and our doctors told us Fiber was good for us...so by buying this product I was making a healthy selection for me and my family.

No one told you that a food or beverage that was not providing you with natural fiber was providing you with Inulin...a substance that the food companies could manipulate into something salty or sweet but it was chemically induced.

## High Fructose Corn Syrup

HFCS was introduced into our food supplies in the mid to late sixties (note: you will see different dates on this but this...but my time period is historically correct)...because of the processing guidelines it leaves trace elements of arsenic and mercury in the finished product. I feel the processing makes HFCS even more of a toxic risk.

Argument for those who disagree—High Fructose Corn Syrup is no different than sugar it has Fructose and Glucose in it just like table sugar. So that can't be the problem...you are too negative toward HFCS.

Argument for those who agree with this statement—look at the research and for those of you against this thought process...provide another answer as to why these health issues increased with the increased consumption of HFCS.

What supports my findings "Cliff Notes Version." Fructose binds with protein, which is processed by the liver (much faster than natural Fructose/Glucose) and is not used in the cells to produce energy. The liver is taxed by the sudden influx of this type of Fructose and the deposits this type of fructose into fat and creates a chronic state of inflammation, as well, in our body.

*Fructose* is not enzymatically regulated and combines with *proteins* haphazardly in the liver, where it is almost entirely processed. Fructose causes seven times as much cell damage as does glucose, because it binds to cellular proteins seven times faster; and it releases 100 times the number of oxygen radicals (such as hydrogen peroxide, which kills everything in sight). Scientific data on fructose says it is one of the most egregious components of the western diet, directly contributing to heart disease and diabetes, and associated with cancer and dementia.

Mercury is toxic in all its forms, and it causes a wide arrange of adverse health effects.

It is high volatile and contamination occurs throughout the process. I only takes a few parts per trillion of species like "ethyl mercury" to induce neurotoxicity.

The Institute for Agriculture and Trade Policy (IATP) study comes on the heels of another study, conducted in 2005 but recently published by the scientific journal. Environmental Health which revealed that nearly fifty (50) percent of commercial high fructose corn syrup (HFCS) same from brand-name food and beverage products test positive for the heavy metal mercury.

Researchers have established the conditions that foster the formation of potentially dangerous levels of a toxic substance in the high fructose corn syrup called: hydroxymethylfurfural (HMF.

GMO's

Genetically modified organisms also known as "GMO's" are now found in as many as 60 to 70 % of the foods in the United States. A genetically modified organism (GMO) is an organism whose genetic material has been altered using genetic engineering techniques.

Genetic modification involves the mutation, insertion, or deletion of genes. When genes are inserted, they usually come from a different species, which is a form of horizontal gene transfer.

246

If it is a genetically modified organism, the DNA has changed and that food now has a different effect on our body and digestive tract.

Argument for those who disagree—the scientific research was done to help people have food. It does not affect us. It has no impact on the human body.

Argument for those who agree with this statement—if you believe that GMO's have no affect on the human body, why do you eat specific things that are good for you?

Any food you ingest theoretically provides fuel and nutritional needs so you can continue to live…if GMO's has no impact on our foods and bodies how do you explain the fact your food provides nutrition…nutrition you get from your food. If you are receiving nourishment from your food than you are also receiving anything negative into your body via the Genetically Modified foods.

What supports my findings: GMO's in our food, exacerbates or creates Food Allergy Symptoms, Bodily Toxicity increases, affects our Reproductive ability, negatively impacts the Digestive System which is tied to our Brain and Immune System and in extreme cases death.

We eat on average 193 pounds of genetically modified foods in a year, at minimum. Yes, you read that right -- 193 pounds!

There are no long-term safety studies in humans. Thus, the long-term health effects are unknown.

Genetically modified crops use more pesticides. Their use has increased by 404 million pounds from 1996 to 2011. And stronger herbicides are needed to counter weed resistance, including 2, 4-D, which is one of the chemicals found in Agent Orange! This is bad for the environment and can't be good for us.

Chemical companies that create GMO seeds -- such as Monsanto -- patent them so farmers have to buy new seeds each year. I just don't think it's right to patent seeds, GMO or otherwise. In addition, think about it, do you really want chemical companies to control our food supply?

It is for these reasons that I avoid genetically modified foods. I hope you consider removing them from your diet as well. Let's use the power we do have -- our dollars -- and avoid GMOs now.

The current crops that are genetically modified are soy, corn, canola, sugar beets, cotton, Hawaiian papaya some zucchini and yellow crookneck squash and alfalfa (which is fed to cattle and not us). Here are some tips to cut GMOs out of your diet.

Before the FDA decided to allow GMOs into food without labeling, FDA scientists had repeatedly warned that GM foods can create unpredictable, hard-to-detect side effects, including allergies, toxins, new diseases, and nutritional problems. They urged long-term safety studies, but were ignored.

This means that long after we stop eating GM foods, we may still have their GM proteins produced continuously inside us. This could mean:

If the antibiotic gene inserted into most GM crops were to transfer, it could create super diseases, resistant to antibiotics

If the gene that creates Bt-toxin in GM corn were to transfer, it might turn our intestinal bacteria into living pesticide factories

Environmental Destruction

Most GMO seeds are genetically engineered to be herbicide tolerant, resistant to insect infestation and disease.

Environmentalists worry that the characteristics of GM crops may encourage farmers to increase their use of herbicides and pesticides, which will raise human consumption of dangerous toxins. GM crops also manufacture their own pesticides, which puts further poisons into humans and soil and may cause unforeseen changes in the environment. Another concern is that toxins contained in the GMO plants may harm other organisms, such as monarch caterpillars, bees and birds. The pesticide found in genetically modified cotton and corn is implicated in the deaths of poultry, cows, horses, sheep and buffalo worldwide.

According to the United States Department of Agriculture, as of 2010, at least 80 percent of corn and approximately 90 percent of soybeans grown in the United States are grown from genetically modified seeds. Genetically modified, or GMO foods, are crops grown from seeds engineered to increase yield and lower production costs. Proponents of GM foods say that the higher yields and improved nutritional content are necessary to ensure adequate food for the world's growing population. Opponents say any claimed benefits of GM foods are unproven, and cite the lack of safety studies and the real and potential dangers to human health and the environment as reasons to ban the products.

## Health Consequences

The rise in autoimmune diseases, infertility, gastrointestinal problems and chronic diseases may be associated with the introduction of GM foods. In a position paper by the American Academy of Environmental Medicine, the authors ask all physicians to consider the role of GM foods in the nation's health crisis, and advise their patients to avoid all GM foods whenever possible. The Academy also recommends a moratorium on GM seeds and calls for immediate independent safety testing and the labeling of all food items containing genetically modified products. As of 2010, the U.S. does not require food manufacturers to identify foodstuffs produced with genetically modified crops.

Genetically modified seeds are a patented product, and in order to purchase the seeds customers must sign an agreement for use with the seed manufacturer.

According to Mike Adams of the Natural News website, Monsanto -- the agritech company that controls approximately 90 percent of the GMO seed market -- prohibits farmers from saving seeds or selling them to other growers. Adams says small, independent farmers, whose crops become contaminated by neighboring GM crops, must pay patent fees or risk being sued.

As the reliance on GM seeds expands worldwide, concerns about food supply and safety continue to escalate. Genetically engineered seeds are identical in structure, and if a problem affects one particular crop, a major crop failure can result.

For example, following the recent failure of three GMO corn crops in three South African provinces, the Africa Centre for Biosecurity has called for an investigation and immediate ban of all GMO food. Corn is a primary source of food for South African nations.

Herbicides and pesticides will raise human consumption of dangerous toxins. GM crops also manufacture their own pesticides, which puts further poisons into humans and soil and may cause unforeseen changes in the environment. Another concern is that toxins contained in the GMO plants may harm other organisms, such as monarch caterpillars, bees and birds. The pesticide found in genetically modified cotton and corn is implicated in the deaths of poultry, cows, horses, sheep and buffalo worldwide.

What we need to do—so we regain our health—reducing the hypersensitive state of our body!

What will it take to correct the chemicals in our food from poisoning us? Eliminate all processed food or make sure the processed food no longer contains chemicals. That labeling is exact, and companies are forthright with their processing procedures so we know what trace elements are in our food.

We need to remove these substances from our diets. Allow our body to return to a non-inflammatory state and then, based on my research, I feel we would see a decrease in the many illnesses that the chemicals have induced or exacerbated.

At the very worst this advise would—provide you with improved health—so, what do you have to lose? (36)

May of 2015 after eliminating all processed foods and any GMO's for nearly 3 years—I no longer test positive for Gluten or Lactose. My body, which had been highjacked by processed food for so long finally started to work the way it was meant to work.

Read, Comprehend, You Decide!

I am sharing articles that come from many research centers. If you read the information that follows the most it can do is educate you or make you curious enough to ask questions—that will lead you to your own results.

Sloan Kettering:

High Fructose Corn Syrup and interesting ways to create pandemics. Part 1

Sweeteners Tags: Corn syrup, Eating, Food, Fructose, Fructose Corn Syrup, Health, HFCS, High-fructose corn syrup, Sugar substitute

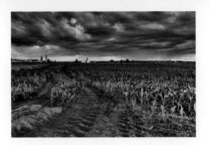

This is to open up an honest debate into the scientific rationale to why High Fructose Corn Syrup may have been a mistake. This is only part 1 of my collection of publically available unedited studies on the subject. Please feel free to re-post, as long as you link me as the original source. This will allow the reader to be aware of future releases as they become available. (36)

## 1. Pancreatic cancers use high fructose corn syrup (HFCS), common in the Western diet to fuel their growth

Pancreatic cancers use high fructose corn syrup (HFCS), common in the Western diet to fuel their growth

All Posts, Consumer Products, Sweeteners  Tags: American Journal of Clinical Nutrition, HFCS, High-fructose corn syrup, Jonsson Comprehensive Cancer Center, National Institutes of Health, Sugar, U.S. News & World Report, United States (37)

Pancreatic cancers use the sugar fructose, very common in the Western diet, to activate a key cellular pathway that drives cell division, helping the cancer to grow more quickly, a study by researchers at UCLA's Jonsson Comprehensive Cancer Center has found.

Although it's widely known that cancers use glucose, a simple sugar, to fuel their growth, this is the first time a link has been shown between fructose and cancer proliferation, said Dr. Anthony Heaney, an associate professor of medicine and neurosurgery, a Jonsson Cancer Center researcher and senior author of the study.

"The bottom line is the modern diet contains a lot of refined sugar including fructose and it's a hidden danger implicated in a lot of modern diseases, such as obesity, diabetes and fatty liver," said Heaney, who also serves as director of the Pituitary Tumor and Neuroendocrine Program at UCLA.

"In this study, we show that cancers can use fructose just as readily as glucose to fuel their growth."

The study appeared in the Aug. 1 issue of the peer-reviewed journal *Cancer Research.*

The source of fructose in the Western diet is high fructose corn syrup (HFCS), a corn-based sweetener that has been on the market since about 1970. HFCS accounts for more than 40 percent of the caloric sweeteners added to foods and beverages, and it is the sole sweetener used in American soft drinks.

Between 1970 and 1990, the consumption of HFCS in the U.S. has increased over 1,000 percent, according to an article in the April 2004 issue of the American Journal of Clinical Nutrition.

Food companies use HFCS – a mixture of fructose and glucose – because it's inexpensive, easy to transport and keeps foods moist. Moreover, because it is so sweet, it's cost effective for companies to use small quantities of HCFS in place of more expensive sweeteners or flavorings.

In his study, Heaney and his team took pancreatic tumors from patients, cultured, and grew the malignant cells in Petri dishes. They then added glucose to one set of cells and fructose to another. Using mass spectrometry, they were able to follow the carbon-labeled sugars in the cells to determine what exactly they were being used for and how.

Heaney found that the pancreatic cancer cells could easily distinguish between glucose and fructose even though they are very similar structurally, and contrary to conventional wisdom, the cancer cells metabolized the sugars in very different ways. In the case of fructose, the pancreatic cancer cells used the sugar in the transketolase-driven non-oxidative pentose phosphate pathway to generate nucleic acids, the building blocks of RNA and DNA, which the cancer cells need to divide and proliferate.

"Traditionally, glucose and fructose have been considered as interchangeable monosaccharide substrates that are similarly metabolized, and little attention has been given to sugars other than glucose," the study states. "However, fructose intake has increased dramatically in recent decades and cellular uptake of glucose and fructose uses distinct transporters ... These findings show that cancer cells can readily metabolize fructose to increase proliferation. They have major significance for cancer patients, given dietary refined fructose consumption."

As in anti-smoking campaigns, a federal effort should be launched to reduce refined fructose intake, Heaney said.

"I think this paper has a lot of public health implications," Heaney said. "Hopefully, at the federal level there will be some effort to step back on the amount of HFCS in our diets."

Heaney said that while this study was done in pancreatic cancer, these finding may not be unique to that cancer type.

Going forward, Heaney and his team are exploring whether it's possible to block the uptake of fructose in the cancer cells with a small molecule, taking away one of the fuels they need to grow. The work is being done in cell lines and in mice, Heaney said.

2. High Fructose Corn Syrup Direct Correlation with Autism in the U.S. – Clinic Epigenetics. 2012

High Fructose Corn Syrup Direct Correlation with Autism in the U.S. – Clinic Epigenetics. 2012

Sweeteners Tags: American Psychiatric Association, ASD, Autism spectrum, Epidemiology of autism, Health, High-fructose corn syrup, Northeastern University, United States.
EEV: Highlights although there are many potential causes

We chose to highlight HFCS, due to its toxin amplification. (38)

1) Ca, Mg and Zn, or losses or displacement of any of these minerals from the consumption of HFCS
2) Mercury (Hg) and fructose may both modulate PON1 activity
3) Mercury (Hg) that may occur from the low Hg concentrations sometimes found in HFCS because of the manufacturing process
4) HFCS, may further enhance the toxic effects of lead (Pb) on cognitive and behavioral development in children

3. Dietary fructose causes liver damage in animal model, study finds
4. Heat forms potentially harmful substance in high-fructose corn syrup: Hydroxymethylfurfural (HMF)

Heat forms potentially harmful substance in high-fructose corn syrup: Hydroxymethylfurfural (HMF) (39)

General Diet, Other Food Additives, Sweeteners   Tags: Agricultural Research Service, Colony collapse disorder, HFCS, High-fructose corn syrup, HMF, Honey bee, Hydroxymethylfurfural, Journal of Agricultural and Food Chemistry, United States

Researchers have established the conditions that foster formation of potentially dangerous levels of a toxic substance in the high-fructose corn syrup (HFCS) often fed to honey bees. Their study, which appears in ACS' bi-weekly *Journal of Agricultural and Food Chemistry*, could also help keep the substance out of soft drinks and dozens of other human foods that contain HFCS. The substance, hydroxymethylfurfural (HMF), forms mainly from heating fructose.

In the new study, Blaise LeBlanc and Gillian Eggleston and colleagues note HFCS's ubiquitous usage as a sweetener in beverages and processed foods. Some commercial beekeepers also feed it to bees to increase reproduction and honey production. When exposed to warm temperatures, HFCS can form HMF and kill honeybees. Some researchers believe that HMF may be a factor in Colony Collapse Disorder, a mysterious disease that has killed at least one-third of the honeybee population in the United States.

The scientists measured levels of HMF in HFCS products from different manufacturers over a period of 35 days at different temperatures. As temperatures rose, levels of HMF increased steadily. Levels jumped dramatically at about 120 degrees Fahrenheit. "The data are important for commercial beekeepers, for manufacturers of HFCS, and for purposes of food storage.

Because HFCS is incorporated as a sweetener in many processed foods, the data from this study are important for human health as well," the report states. It adds that studies have linked HMF to DNA damage in humans. In addition, HMF breaks down in the body to other substances potentially more harmful than HMF.

5. US researchers find traces of toxic mercury in high-fructose corn syrup

Eating Foods High in Fructose from Added Sugars Linked to Hypertension

Fructose-sweetened but not glucose-sweetened beverages can adversely affect both sensitivity to the hormone insulin and how the body handles fats

HFCS triggering type 2 diabetes epidemic

High Fructose Sets Table for Weight Gain Without Warning: Leptin Resistance

High-fructose corn syrup sugar makes maturing human fat cells fatter, less insulin-sensitive

Increased dietary fructose (high fructose corn syrup) linked to elevated uric acid levels and lower liver energy stores

Princeton researchers find that high-fructose corn syrup prompts considerably more weight gain

Excessive fructose may be making 'spoiled appetites' a thing of the past In "Sweeteners"

Excessive fructose may be making 'spoiled appetites' a thing of the past In "Sweeteners"

Princeton researchers find that high-fructose corn syrup prompts considerably more weight gain: rats became obese by drinking high-fructose corn syrup, but not by drinking sucrose

University Of Southern California and Oxford Researchers Find High Fructose Corn Syrup-Global Prevalence of Diabetes Link!

International analysis finds that countries using high fructose corn syrup in their food supply have a 20 percent higher prevalence of type 2 diabetes

LOS ANGELES AND OXFORD, U.K. — a new study by University of Southern California (USC) and University of Oxford researchers indicates that large amounts of high fructose corn syrup (HFCS) found in national food supplies across the world may be one explanation for the rising global epidemic of type 2 diabetes and resulting higher health care costs. (40)

The study reports that countries that use HFCS in their food supply had a 20 percent higher prevalence of diabetes than countries that did not use HFCS.

257

The analysis also revealed that HFCS's association with the "significantly increased prevalence of diabetes" occurred independent of total sugar intake and <u>obesity</u> levels.

The article, "High Fructose Corn Syrup and Diabetes Prevalence: A Global Perspective," is published in the journal *Global Public Health.*

"HFCS appears to pose a serious public health problem on a global scale," said principal study author Michael I. Goran, professor of preventive medicine, director of the Childhood Obesity Research Center and co-director of the Diabetes and Obesity Research Institute at the Keck School of Medicine at USC."
The study adds to a growing body of scientific literature that indicates HFCS consumption may result in negative health consequences distinct from and more deleterious than natural sugar."

The paper reports that out of 42 countries studied, the United States has the highest per capita consumption of HFCS at a rate of 25 kilograms, or 55 pounds, per year. The second highest is Hungary, with an annual rate of 16 kilograms, or 46 pounds, per capita.

Canada, Slovakia, Bulgaria, Belgium, Argentina, Korea, Japan, and Mexico are also relatively high HFCS consumers. Germany, Poland, Greece, Portugal, Egypt, Finland, and Serbia are among the lowest HFCS consumers. Countries with per capita consumption of less than 0.5 kilogram per year include Australia, China, Denmark, France, India, Ireland, Italy, Sweden, the United Kingdom, and Uruguay.

Countries with higher use of HFCS had an average prevalence of type 2 diabetes of 8 percent compared to 6.7 percent in countries not using HFCS.

"This research suggests that HFCS can increase the risk of type 2 diabetes, which is one of the most common causes of death in the world today," said study co-author Professor Stanley Ulijaszek, director of the Institute of Social and Cultural Anthropology at the University of Oxford.

The article proposes that this link is probably driven by higher amounts of fructose in foods and beverages made with HFCS. Fructose and glucose are both found in ordinary sugar (sucrose) in equal amounts, but HFCS has a greater proportion of fructose.

The higher fructose content makes HFCS sweeter and provides processed foods with greater stability and better appearance because of the more consistent browning color when foods made with higher fructose are baked.

In a previous related study, the authors found that the fructose content in some U.S.-produced soft drinks, especially the most popular, was about 20 percent higher than expected, suggesting that some manufacturers might be using HFCS with more fructose than previously estimated.

Such differences could "potentially be driving up fructose consumption in countries that use HFCS," the researchers said. The study notes the difficulty in determining the actual amount of fructose in foods and beverages made with HFCS because of "a lack of industry disclosure on food labels."

Growing evidence reveals that the body metabolizes fructose differently from glucose. Among other things, fructose metabolism occurs independently of insulin, primarily in the liver where it may be readily converted to fat, which likely contributes to non-alcoholic fatty liver disease, a condition on the rise in Hispanics in the U.S. and Mexico.

"Most populations have an almost insatiable appetite for sweet foods, but regrettably our metabolism has not evolved sufficiently to be able to process the fructose from high fructose corn syrup in the quantities that some people are consuming it," said Ulijaszek. "Although this syrup can be found in many of our processed foods and drinks, this varies enormously from country to country."

The U.S. is the single largest consumer of high fructose corn syrup. By the late 1990s, HFCS made up 40 percent of all caloric sweeteners and was the predominant sweetener in soft drinks sold in the U.S.

However, since 2008, exports of HFCS from the U.S. to Mexico increased "exponentially" after trade restrictions were removed, the researchers said. They call for updated public health strategies requiring better labeling of fructose and HFCS content in processed foods.

To explain the varying degrees of HFCS consumption in the European Union, the researchers note that trade and agricultural policies set quotas for HFCS production, and while some countries, such as Sweden and the U.K., do not take their assigned quotas, other countries, such as Hungary and Slovakia, are able to purchase extra quotas from countries that do not accept them.

The findings of the paper thus have important implications for global trade policies that may affect public health.

"If HFCS is a risk factor for diabetes—one of the world's most serious chronic diseases—then we need to rewrite national dietary guidelines and review agriculture trade policies," said Tim Lobstein, director of policy for the International Association for the Study of Obesity. "HFCS will join Trans fats and salt as ingredients to avoid, and foods should carry warning labels." (41)

Background Information:

Sources of data in the ecological analysis include the Global Burden of Metabolic Risk Factors Collaborating Group (BMI), International Diabetes Federation Diabetes Atlas (prevalence), and the FAOSTAT, a statistical website maintained by the Food and Agriculture Organization of the United Nations (food availability).

People suffering from type 2 diabetes have high blood glucose due to insulin resistance. Though the exact cause of Type II diabetes is not known, studies frequently attribute it to excess weight and lack of activity. Recent research estimates that 6.4 percent of the world population is diabetic and by 2030, the estimate will increase to 7.7 percent, with developing countries seeing the highest increases. Wider acceptance of processed foods with higher levels of refined carbohydrates, especially sugar, is considered by some experts to be a reason. Complications from type 2 diabetes include blindness, dementia, gum disease, cardiovascular disease, and an increase in lower limb amputations. Those with type 2 diabetes typically have a 10-year shorter life span than the general population.

## Cannabis Less Addicting Than High Fructose Corn Syrup!

The following article By Walking Times written by Marco Tores, Prevent Disease March 2014

There are so many addictive substances in our society that we humans love to portray as evil. We label them as such because of our tendencies and repetition towards anything that is considered to have negative consequences.

We are never to be accountable for our actions or behavior–it's always the drug or plant that is responsible and at fault for all our problems. Out of all the addictive substances we love to demonize, guess which one is rarely if ever a type of substance dependent drug?

In the mental health profession's "bible," the _Diagnostic and Statistical Manual of Mental Disorders_, a diagnosis of cannabis dependence (a type of substance dependence) requires a person to meet a specific set of criteria.

A number of investigators have addressed this issue and found that, unlike drugs such as crack, cocaine, or even nicotine, only a very small percentage of those who try marijuana will ever become addicted. On the following list, marijuana does not even come close to the substance and dependence abuse rates of the others listed.

Many factors determine whether you'll become addicted to a drug: your genetic makeup, social history, the drugs your friends take, how much money you make. However, the chemical makeup of drugs guarantees that certain drugs are more addictive than others.

A team of researchers led by Professor David Nutt of London's Imperial College once set out to determine which drugs were most harmful based on their addictive properties (the resulting article suggested that alcohol and tobacco are more harmful than cannabis and ecstasy, and led to Nutt being _fired_ as the UK's top drug adviser).

Dutch scientists replicated the London study and devised a "dependency rating" that measured addictive potency of the biggest drugs out there on a precisely calibrated scale of 0-to-3.

The Top 13 Most Addictive Substances

10. GHB-Dependence Rating (out of 3) 1.71

Last on the list and being, the weakest in terms of dependence is a depressant and club drug that may itself be a neurotransmitter.

It has cross-tolerance with alcohol–if you drink regularly, you'll need to ingest more GHB to get high–as well as a short half-life in the body and a brutal withdrawal syndrome that causes insomnia, anxiety, dizziness and vomiting.

The combination is nasty: Take a lot of GHB to make up for your tolerance to alcohol and you could be hooked.

### 9. Benzodiazepines - Dependence Rating: 1.89

There is a reason your doctor will tell you to taper off these prescription anti-anxiety drugs (Valium, Xanax, Klonopin, et al) after taking them for a while. Each one increase the effectiveness of a brain chemical called GABA, which reduces the excitability of many other neurons and decreases anxiety. Because benzodiazepines cause rapid tolerance, quitting cold turkey causes a multi-symptom withdrawal that includes irritability, anxiety and panic attacks–enough to make just about anybody fall right back into benzo's comforting arms.

### 8. Amphetamines – Dependence Rating: 1.95

Adderall users beware: Regular amphetamine (classified as pure or blended dextroamphetamine without methamphetamine, and including Adderall, Dexedrine, and Desoxyn) might not be quite as addictive as meth, but because it acts on the same reward circuit, it still causes rapid tolerance and desire for more if used regularly or in high doses.

Quitting cold turkey can cause severe depression and anxiety, as well as extreme fatigue–and you can guess what extreme fatigue makes you crave.

### 7. Cocaine – Dependence Rating: 2.13

Cocaine use has decreased dramatically but it is another drug that costs families, and our society as a whole. It is a heavily habit forming drug. While it does enter the list as slightly less addictive than Nicotine and Caffeine, the effects of Cocaine's (and heroin's) use are far more serious.

Drug rehab programs list cocaine as one of the top addictions they face daily. Cocaine prevents the re-absorption of dopamine in the brain's reward areas. After you use enough blow, your brain reduces the number of dopamine receptors in this region, figuring it already has plenty of it. You can see where this is going.

Because there are now fewer receptors, stopping the drug makes you crave it–after all, the body needs its dopamine. Cocaine doesn't destroy dopamine neurons like methamphetamine, which makes its effect less powerfully addictive, but the fast method of use (snorting), short high (less than an hour) and rapid tolerance put it in the top ten.

## 6. Alcohol – Dependence Rating: 2.13

Because alcohol is legal and often consumed in social settings, alcohol addiction is complicated. Nevertheless, as an addictive agent, it's remarkably simple–and effective.

Alcohol's withdrawal syndrome is so severe that it can cause death, and its effects on the brain's reward system cause well-documented and intense craving in heavy drinkers. Regardless of the mechanism, 17.9 million Americans (7% of the US population) were classified as being addicted to or abusing alcohol in 2010. It acts as a relaxant, causing the user to feel more comfortable in an environment and leading to increased sociability. However, in larger doses alcohol begins to have serious detrimental effects on a person's health.

Addiction to alcohol, as well as being expensive, can lead to serious liver problems, diabetes, cancer and heart problems.

Short-term effects of alcohol include dehydration, alcohol poisoning, and intoxication.

## 5. Crystal Meth – Dependence Rating: 2.24

According to some research, Crystal Meth is regarded as one of the most addictive recreational drugs in existence. Directly mimicking a natural neurotransmitter "teaches" your brain to want a drug–that's how nicotine and heroin work. Crystal methamphetamine takes it to the next level: it imitates the reward chemical dopamine and the alertness chemical norepinephrine, causing your neurons to release more of both–all the while training your brain to want them more.

What's worse, the drug can damage dopamine- and norepinephrine-releasing neurons, which leads to a drastic decrease in their production, thereby making you crave more meth. It's an addict's nightmare and a marketer's dream. Crystal Meth is used to make the user feel more alert, heightening their awareness and bringing on an intense feeling of exhilaration. Meth also has the ability to keep the user awake for many hours. The drug can be taken in a variety of ways, but the most common method is via injection as this is the fastest acting way of taking the drug. Crystal meth addiction can lead to a hideous array of effects, including violent mood swings, short-term memory loss, damaging of the nervous system and even death.

### 4. Methadone – Dependence Rating: 2.68

In a clinical setting, tolerance to this drug is actually considered a good thing when treating a heroin addiction.

A junky being treated with methadone will quickly become resistant to its euphoric effects and use it to keep heroin withdrawal symptoms at bay. The problem is this: tolerance to methadone is a sign of an addiction to methadone.

### 3. Nicotine – Dependence Rating: 2.82

Though nicotine doesn't cause the rush of heroin or crack, it's biologically similar in a crucial way: it mimics a common neurotransmitter–so well that scientists named one of the acetylcholine receptors after it.

Nicotine is considered one of the most addictive drugs of all time. Although studies vary, it is generally believed that well over 30% of those individuals who use nicotine for a period of time become addicted.

That is a high number considering the availability of the product, the manner in which it is marketed towards young people, and the deadly consequences of a lifetime of use.

Smoking regularly reduces the number and sensitivity of these "nicotinic" receptors, and requires that the user keep ingesting nicotine just to maintain normal brain function.

There are a shocking 50,000,000 nicotine addicts in the US, and <u>one in every five</u> deaths nationwide are the result of smoking.

## 2. Crack Cocaine – Dependence Rating: 2.82

Crack cocaine is a cheaper form of the purer Cocaine drug, and is far more dangerous as a result. It is watered down and 'cooked' cocaine, and is usually smoked in a pipe or (rarely) injected intravenously. Although crack cocaine and powder cocaine have similar chemical compositions and effects, smoking processed crack causes a faster, higher rush that lasts for less time (about 10 minutes, versus 15-30 for powder cocaine).

Crack brings on an increased sense of confidence, awareness, and euphoria, while simultaneously causing a dilation of the pupils and constriction of the blood vessels.

Crack cocaine is so addictive because of the incredible low experienced after the short period of euphoria, during which users can feel depressed and tired and are easily irritated or angered. Crack addicts therefore continually seek new ways to feed their addiction to avoid the low, which comes after crack usage.

The intensity of the high combined with the efficient method of ingestion smoking is the big reasons why addiction rates are dramatically higher for crack than they are for snorted powder. In 2010, there were an estimated 500,000 active crack cocaine addicts in the United States.

## 1. Heroin – Dependence Rating: 2.89

Although one-hundred years ago Heroin was used for a variety of medicinal purposes, the medical community in all their infinite wisdom woke up to the realization that people were becoming addicted in record numbers.

Heroin is one of the most common recreational drugs in the world, with an estimated 50 million regular uses of the drug worldwide.

As an opiate, it affects opioid receptors throughout the body and mimics endorphins, reducing pain and causing pleasure.

Areas of the brain involved in reward processing and learning are stocked with tons of these opioid receptors, so when you inject heroin, you are training your brain to make you crave it. Pair that with nasty withdrawal symptoms and high fat solubility (which allows it to get into your brain quickly), and you have the most addictive drug in the world. An estimated 281,000 people received treatment for heroin addiction in the US in 2003, and according to the National Institute on Drug Addiction, a full 23 percent of people who have ever used heroin become addicts.

Heroin is usually injected directly into the blood stream, though it can also be snorted or smoked by its users.

Continuous usage of Heroin can lead to collapsed veins, heart disease and decreased liver function. Heroin addicts also typically bare numerous hideous abscesses on their skin, as well as scars where they have repeatedly injected themselves over the course of their addiction.

## Caffeine

Although not on David Nutt's list, Caffeine is also considered to be on par if not a greater addictive drug than amphetamines and much higher in dependence than marijuana. Caffeine would have ranked high on this list if it were included in the study because almost 30% of casual users become addicted. This stimulant is found is so many things we consume every day that you have to look hard to find a product without it.

Caffeine is a commonplace central nervous system stimulant drug, which occurs in nature as part of the coffee, tea, yerba mate and some other plants.

However, it also an <u>unnatural additive</u> in many consumer products, most notably beverages advertised as energy drinks. Caffeine is also added to sodas such as Coca-Cola and Pepsi, where on the ingredients listing, it is designated as a flavoring agent.

Roland Griffiths, a professor in the departments of psychiatry and neuroscience at the Johns Hopkins School of Medicine, said that studies had demonstrated that people who take in a minimum of 100 mg of caffeine per day (about the amount in one cup of coffee) can acquire a physical dependence that would trigger withdrawal symptoms that include headaches, muscle pain and stiffness, lethargy, nausea, vomiting, depressed mood, and marked irritability.

## High Fructose Corn Syrup Is Causing Addiction Similar To Cocaine

Results <u>presented at the 2013 Canadian Neuroscience Meeting</u> shows that high-fructose corn syrup (HFCS) can cause behavioral reactions similar to those produced by drugs of abuse such as cocaine. These results, presented by addiction expert Francesco Leri, Associate Professor of Neuroscience, and Applied Cognitive Science at the University of Guelph, suggest food addiction could explain, at least partly, the current global obesity epidemic partly caused by these ingredients.

Cannabis/Marijuana:

To the shock of many who study drug dependence, marijuana rarely ranks compared to others dependent drugs. Government studies will often focus on recreational use rather than dependence, but there is a big difference.

Is Sugar Toxic?

New York Times Article on Robert Lustig Sugar

Please Note: this article contains Pros and Cons on both Sugar and HFCS. The article is not in its entirety. The study was done prior to 2008. (42)

On May 26, 2009, Robert Lustig gave a lecture called "Sugar: The Bitter Truth," which was posted on YouTube the following July. Since then, it has been viewed well over 800,000 times, gaining new viewers at a rate of about 50,000 per month, remarkable numbers for a 90-minute discussion of the nuances of fructose biochemistry and human physiology.

*What the average American consumes in added sugars: both Sugar and High Fructose Corn Syrup.*

High Fructose Corn Syrup Consumption (2008)

One Day 1.4 ounces=Shot glass

One Week 9.8 ounces=Large Glass

One Month 5.3 Cups=Pitcher

One Year 4 Gallons = Bucket

Lifetime 313 Gallons= Hot Tub

*Sugar Consumption (2008)*

One Day 11.9 teaspoons = Small Trowel

One Week 1.7 Cups = Large Trowel

One Month 7.5 Cups= Large Plant Pot

One Year 45.3 Pounds = Wheel Barrow

Lifetime 3, 550 pounds= Large Waste Container

It doesn't hurt Lustig's cause that he is a compelling public speaker. His critics argue that what makes him compelling is his practice of taking suggestive evidence and insisting that it's incontrovertible. Lustig certainly doesn't dabble in shades of gray. Sugar is not just an empty calorie, he says; its effect on us is much more insidious. "It's not about the calories," he says. "It has nothing to do with the calories. It's a poison by itself."

If Lustig is right, then our excessive consumption of sugar is the primary reason that the numbers of obese and diabetic Americans have skyrocketed in the past 30 years. However, his argument implies more than that. If Lustig is right, it would mean that sugar is also the likely dietary cause of several other chronic ailments widely considered to be diseases of Western lifestyles — heart disease, hypertension and many common cancers among them

The number of viewers Lustig has attracted suggests that people are paying attention to his argument.

When I set out to interview public health authorities and researchers for this article, they would often initiate the interview with some variation of the comment "surely you've spoken to Robert Lustig," not because Lustig has done any of the key research on sugar himself, which he hasn't, but because he's willing to insist publicly and unambiguously, when most researchers are not, that sugar is a toxic substance that people abuse. In Lustig's view, sugar should be thought of, like cigarettes and alcohol, as something that's killing us.

This brings us to the salient question: Can sugar possibly be as bad as Lustig says it is?

It's one thing to suggest, as most nutritionists will, that a healthful diet include more fruits and vegetables, and maybe less fat, red meat and salt, or less of everything.

It's entirely different to claim that one particularly cherished aspect of our diet might not just be an unhealthful indulgence but actually be toxic, that when you make your children a birthday cake or give them lemonade on a hot summer day, you may be doing them more harm than good, despite all the love that goes with it. Suggesting that sugar might kill us is what zealots do.

However, Lustig, who has genuine expertise, has accumulated, and synthesized a mass of evidence, which he finds compelling enough to convict sugar.

His critics consider that evidence insufficient, but there's no way to know who might be right, or what must be done to find out, without discussing it.

If I didn't buy this argument myself, I wouldn't be writing about it here. In addition, I also have a disclaimer to acknowledge. I've spent much of the last decade doing journalistic research on diet and chronic disease — some of the more contrarian findings, on dietary fat, appeared in this magazine —– and I have come to conclusions similar to Lustig's.

The history of the debate over the health effects of sugar has gone on far longer than you might imagine.

It is littered with erroneous statements and conclusions because even the supposed authorities had no true understanding of what they were talking about. They didn't know, quite literally, what they meant by the word "sugar" and therefore what the implications were.

So let's start by clarifying a few issues, beginning with Lustig's use of the word "sugar" to mean both sucrose — beet and cane sugar, whether white or brown — *and* high-fructose corn syrup.

This is a critical point, particularly because high-fructose corn syrup has indeed become "the flashpoint for everybody's distrust of processed foods," says Marion Nestle, a New York University nutritionist and the author of "Food Politics."

This development is recent and borders on humorous. In the early *(note…this date is not correct…it was in the late 1960's)* 1980's, high-fructose corn syrup replaced sugar in sodas and other products in part because refined sugar then had the reputation as a generally noxious nutrient. ("Villain in Disguise?" asked a headline in this paper in 1977, before answering in the affirmative.) High-fructose corn syrup was portrayed by the food industry as a healthful alternative, and that's how the public perceived it.

It was also cheaper than sugar, which didn't hurt its commercial prospects. Now the tide is rolling the other way, and refined sugar is making a commercial comeback as the supposedly healthful alternative to this noxious corn-syrup stuff. "Industry after industry is replacing their product with sucrose and advertising it as such — 'No High-Fructose Corn Syrup,' " Nestle notes.

The question, then, isn't whether high-fructose corn syrup is worse than sugar; it's what do they do to us, and how do they do it?

The conventional wisdom has long been that the worst that can be said about sugars of any kind is that they cause tooth decay and represent "empty calories" that we eat in excess because they taste so good.

By this logic, sugar-sweetened beverages (or H.F.C.S.-sweetened beverages, as the Sugar Association prefers they are called) are bad for us not because there's anything particularly toxic about the sugar they contain but just because people consume too many of them.

Those organizations that now advise us to cut down on our sugar consumption — the Department of Agriculture, for instance, in its recent Dietary Guidelines for Americans, or the American Heart Association in guidelines released in September 2009 (of which Lustig was a co-author) — do so for this reason. Refined sugar and H.F.C.S. don't come with any protein, vitamins, minerals, antioxidants or fiber, and so they either displace other more nutritious elements of our diet or are eaten over and above what we need to sustain our weight, and this is why we get fatter.

Whether the empty-calories argument is true, it's certainly convenient. It allows everyone to assign blame for obesity and, by extension, diabetes — two conditions so intimately linked that some authorities have taken to calling them "diabesity" — to overeating of all foods, or under exercising, because a calorie is a calorie. "

Lustig's argument, however, is not about the consumption of empty calories — and biochemists have made the same case previously, though not so publicly. It is that sugar has unique characteristics, specifically in the way the human body metabolizes the fructose in it that may make it singularly harmful, at least if consumed in sufficient quantities.

The fructose component of sugar and H.F.C.S. is metabolized primarily by the liver, while the glucose from sugar and starches is metabolized by every cell in the body.

Consuming sugar (fructose and glucose) means more work for the liver than if you consumed the same number of calories of starch (glucose).

And if you take that sugar in liquid form — soda or fruit juices — the fructose and glucose will hit the liver more quickly than if you consume them, say, in an apple (or several apples, to get what researchers would call the equivalent dose of sugar). The speed with which the liver has to do its work will also affect how it metabolizes the fructose and glucose.

The last time an agency of the federal government looked into the question of sugar and health in any detail was in 2005, in a report by the Institute of Medicine, a branch of the National Academies. The authors of the report acknowledged that plenty of evidence suggested that sugar could increase the risk of heart disease and diabetes — even raising LDL cholesterol, known as the "bad cholesterol"—– but did not consider the research to be definitive. There was enough ambiguity, they concluded, that they couldn't even set an upper limit on how much sugar constitutes too much.

The question is always at what dose does a substance go from being harmless to harmful? How much do we have to consume before this happens?

When Glinsmann and his F.D.A. co-authors decided no conclusive evidence demonstrated harm at the levels of sugar then being consumed, they estimated those levels at 40 pounds per person per year beyond what we might get naturally in fruits and vegetables — 40 pounds per person per year of "added sugars" as nutritionists now call them. This is 200 calories per day of sugar, which is less than the amount in a can and a half of Coca-Cola or two cups of apple juice. If that were indeed all we consume, most nutritionists today would be delighted, including Lustig.

But 40 pounds per year happened to be 35 pounds less than what Department of Agriculture analysts said we were consuming at the time — 75 pounds per person per year — and the U.S.D.A. estimates are typically considered to be the most reliable. By the early 2000s, according to the U.S.D.A., we had increased our consumption to more than 90 pounds per person per year.

This correlation between sugar consumption and diabetes is what defense attorneys call circumstantial evidence. It's more compelling than it otherwise might be, though, because the last time sugar consumption jumped markedly in this country, it was also associated with a diabetes epidemic.

Until Lustig came along, the last time an academic forcefully put forward the sugar-as-toxin thesis was in the 1970s, when John Yudkin, a leading authority on nutrition in the United Kingdom, published a polemic on sugar called "Sweet and Dangerous."

What has changed since then, other than Americans getting fatter and more diabetic? It wasn't so much that researchers learned anything particularly new about the effects of sugar or high-fructose corn syrup in the human body.

Rather the context of the science changed: physicians and medical authorities came to accept the idea that a condition known as metabolic syndrome is a major, if not *the* major, risk factor for heart disease and diabetes.

The Centers for Disease Control and Prevention now estimate that some 75 million Americans have metabolic syndrome. For those who have heart attacks, metabolic syndrome will very likely be the reason.

The first symptom doctors are told to look for in diagnosing metabolic syndrome is an expanding waistline. This means that if you're overweight, there's a good chance you have metabolic syndrome, and this is why you're more likely to have a heart attack or become diabetic (or both) than someone who's not.

Although lean individuals, too, can have metabolic syndrome, and they are at greater risk of heart disease and diabetes than lean individuals without it are.

Having metabolic syndrome is another way of saying that the cells in your body are actively ignoring the action of the hormone insulin — a condition known technically as being insulin-resistant. Because insulin resistance and metabolic syndrome still get remarkably little attention in the press (certainly compared with cholesterol), let me explain the basics.

You secrete insulin in response to the foods you eat — particularly the carbohydrates — to keep blood sugar in control after a meal.

When your cells are resistant to insulin, your body (your pancreas, to be precise) responds to rising blood sugar by pumping out more and more insulin. Eventually the pancreas can no longer keep up with the demand or it gives in to what diabetologists call "pancreatic exhaustion." Now your blood sugar will rise out of control, and you have diabetes.

Not everyone with insulin resistance becomes diabetic; some continue to secrete enough insulin to overcome their cells' resistance to the hormone. However, having chronically elevated insulin levels has harmful effects of its own — heart disease, for one.

This raises two obvious questions. The first is what sets off metabolic syndrome to begin with, which is another way of asking, What causes the initial insulin resistance? There are several hypotheses, but researchers who study the mechanisms of insulin resistance now think that a likely cause is the accumulation of fat in the liver.

When studies have been done trying to answer this question in humans, says Varman Samuel, who studies insulin resistance at Yale School of Medicine, the correlation between liver fat and insulin resistance in patients, lean or obese, is "remarkably strong."
What it looks like, Samuel says, is that "when you deposit fat in the liver, that's when you become insulin-resistant."

That raises the other obvious question: What causes the liver to accumulate fat in humans?

A common assumption is that simply getting fatter leads to a fatty liver, but this does not explain fatty liver in lean people. Some of it could be attributed to genetic predisposition. Nevertheless, harking back to Lustig, there's also the very real possibility that it is caused by sugar.
As it happens, metabolic syndrome and insulin resistance are the reasons that many of the researchers today studying fructose became interested in the subject to begin with.

If you want to cause insulin resistance in laboratory rats, says Gerald Reaven, the Stanford University diabetologist who did much of the pioneering work on the subject, feeding those diets that are mostly fructose is an easy way to do it. It's a "very obvious, very dramatic" effect, Reaven says.

By the early 2000s, researchers studying fructose metabolism had established certain findings unambiguously and had well-established biochemical explanations for what was happening.

Feed animals enough pure fructose or enough sugar, and their livers convert the fructose into fat — the saturated fatty acid, palmitate, to be precise, that supposedly gives us heart disease when we eat it, by raising LDL cholesterol. The fat accumulates in the liver, and insulin resistance and metabolic syndrome follow.

Michael Pagliassotti, a Colorado State University biochemist who did many of the relevant animal studies in the late 1990s, says these changes can happen in as little as a week if the animals are fed sugar or fructose in huge amounts — 60 or 70 percent of the calories in their diets.

They can take several months if the animals are fed something closer to what humans (in America) actually consume — around 20 percent of the calories in their diet. Stop feeding them the sugar, in either case, the fatty liver promptly goes away, and with it the insulin resistance.

Similar effects can be shown in humans, although the researchers doing this work typically did the studies with only fructose — as Luc Tappy did in Switzerland or Peter Havel and Kimber Stanhope did at the University of California, Davis — and pure fructose is not the same thing as sugar or high-fructose corn syrup.

When Tappy fed his human subjects the equivalent of the fructose in 8 to 10 cans of Coke or Pepsi a day — a "pretty high dose," he says — – their livers would start to become insulin-resistant, and their triglycerides would go up in just a few days. With lower doses, Tappy says, just as in the animal research, the same effects would appear, but it would take longer, a month or more.

This is why the research reviews on the subject invariably conclude that more research is necessary to establish at what dose sugar and high-fructose corn syrup start becoming what Lustig calls toxic.

"There is clearly a need for intervention studies," as Tappy recently phrased it in the technical jargon of the field, "in which the fructose intake of high-fructose consumers is reduced to better delineate the possible pathogenic role of fructose.

At present, short-term-intervention studies, however, suggest that a high-fructose intake consisting of soft drinks, sweetened juices or bakery products can increase the risk of metabolic and cardiovascular diseases."

In simpler language—how much of this stuff do we have to eat or drink, and for how long, before it does to us what it does to laboratory rats? In addition—is that amount—more than we're already consuming? **Note this was written prior to 2008.**

## My Challenge to You– Patient, Parent, or Spouse!

Throughout the book and particularly in this chapter I have given you information from solid sources. Now it is time for you to become involved and make your own decisions.

I would ask you to think of one thing. Those research papers that site that HFCS and GMO's are harming us can also substantiate the rise in diseases in direct correlation to the consumption of these items.

If you look at the other side of this debate – how do they explain the rise of these diseases during the same period of consumption of the products…if it is not HFCS and GMO's creating the issues then how do they explain the findings?

I have had many people argue that they could find information that states that HFCS and GMO's are fine and the rest of us are crazy— but not one person could provide an answer to the increase in the diseases and why it correlates with the use of HFCS and GMO's.

❧

The doctor I dedicated my book to provided me with a list of foods that I shouldn't eat 25 to 30 years ago…I pulled out the list from a box and the paper is yellowed the type is faded but the information…well that is still the same. I'm just sorry I didn't keep the list where I could have used it! It took almost dying to remember something I had already been taught!

When I first became ill, I had no idea that medication and/or surgery was not the normal process of treatment.

As days turned into weeks and weeks into months and I had not improved, I started to doubt that anyone was really trying to help me. Much later, I realized I was not alone regarding my opinion of the Medical Profession. The GI Specialists are no longer asking the how and why and we end up in this wasteland of non-specific diagnoses that leave us sick and over-medicated.

It has been made clear that GI specialists know that Fructose and Fructose Malabsorption exist but the majority of them are not treating the patient with the proper protocol. That would be nutrition and diet. They can't help their patients until they move from the medications and look at the cause of the issue.

I went on line to find literally thousands of individuals that belong to groups who have given up hope that their doctor will ever be able to help them. They are moving away from conventional medicine in droves because they are desperate for help. These disgruntled and frustrated patients are seeking help from natural and homeopathic sources due to the growing frustration with their GI Specialists.

What perplexes me is that the medical industry doesn't see the problem.

I went from being in pain 24 hours a day and it lasted for 2 ½ years without one doctor, ER personal or specialist recognizing that I had a very real health issue and they were doing nothing to help me. If anything, they made it worse.

I read how frustrated these people are and instead of turning to their doctor they now turn to groups that can have as many as 13,000 members for help

Their complaints:

- IBS
- Leaky Gut
- SIBO
- Candida
- Fructose Malabsorption
- Hereditary Fructose Intolerance
- Colitis
- Crohn's Disease
- Gastritis
- Lactose Intolerance
- Gluten Intolerance
- Celiac
- Bowel Disease/Distress
- Misc. Tummy Problems.

In addition, several more issues that I haven't listed.

I read the same complaints and symptoms repeatedly and many of the symptoms overlap from one health issue to another. When will we get research from medical science and not the medical industry that will provide us with a trusted and very concise path to follow?

I know what worked for me and I trust every word of my research because my life literally depended on the outcome being accurate. I worked for a long time to fine tune what works for 'me" as a patient since I was diagnosed with HFI.

I can't guarantee that my information will provide the same level of success for everyone because there are variables I can't control. It will depend on how dedicated you are to following the food selections—as to your outcome.

I have read too much convoluted information on-line which only makes the confusion worse. It is very difficult to cut to the chase and find what the answer is for each person.

I stand firm that my research will make you feel better...nothing I have shared or suggested will hurt you.

Several people are suffering from multiply issues and many of the issues can co-exist so what is the best path for them? One diet will contradict the other diet and I see no end of the confusion and frustration for these individuals. My suggestion would be that you are tested for all of the intolerances and start with the issue you seem be the most susceptible to...one day at a time!

This is my challenge to each doctor!

Find the how and why for the sake of all of us!

Demand research from medical research facilities and not medical industry facilities. We deserve your complete attention and nothing less.

Therefore, all respected doctor's the ball is back in your court and you need to start finding solutions that people will once again trust.

I know not all issues can be handled with diet and the proper nutrition, medication, and surgery sometimes might be the answer but please make sure it is the correct solution for each individual who has trusted you with their health and their life.

A spoonful of sugar doesn't help the medicine in the case of a malabsorption problem.

Make sure you read labels on the medication you are taking. Whether prescribed or over the counter. Many medications have sugar and or HFCS in them so the flavor is more palatable for the patient.

You must keep in mind that toothpaste, mouthwash, vitamins, probiotics, Milk of Magnesium, cough-drops, cough-syrup, breath mints and even the bowel prep for your colonoscopy has sugar in it and if you have a malabsorption to fructose all of these products will aggravate your health while you think it may be helping.

The ingredients are on-line and often the sugar and fructose is hidden by stating the term flavoring or another very vague listing. Be responsible and perform due diligence on your medications.

Obviously, if you are going to be tested for a Malabsorption issue then you know you will be given a prep that contains fructose and can anticipate an issue. However, many times, you're blind-sided and the result is not a pleasant one.

If you are in the hospital—unbelievably—this is not a "fructose" well of knowledge when it comes to feeding you. Don't eat the Jell-O!

If you are admitted to the hospital, have meals prepared by someone who really understands what a Fructose Malabsorption patient can eat.

Check out all liquid supplements such as Glucerna, Boost, Ensure and others as many have HFCS or sugar which will have a negative impact on a Fructose Malabsorption individual.

I have provided you with everything you need to improve your health and I can personally attest to everything written in this book. What I promised you in the beginning I have delivered. I have explained how to identify fructose/HFCS; I have provided a thorough understanding of HFCS, as well as, guidance for you in order to eradicate HFCS from your diet.

What would it mean to you if you were no longer hampered by your health issues? How would you like to look and feel younger? How much better off would you be if you had mental clarity, increased energy, and less anxiety? Those changes are possible now.

### Resources to Change Your Life!

1. Follow the Fructose-Specific Food Chart this will help you to Identify where Fructose is in your foods
2. Educated yourself on your health issues
3. By following the Fructose Specific Food Charts and information I have provided to you in this book will provide you with the tools to Eradicate Fructose form your diet!

By following the information in this book and the three steps above, it will help you lose weight, increase your energy, decrease your depression, eliminate bloating and gas and your intestinal tract will be well on the way to good health!

But—it is not a magic pill or product! It takes you investing in your health and that of your families to improve your current health issues.

There are no cures of the illnesses I have listed but you will find a way to manage your condition while improving the areas of your life you can control.

Make a conscious decision to remove processed food from your diet. Eating fresh or Organic is only on an average of $5.00 per person per day more than what you are paying for processed food.

Remember how important your Digestive Tract is to your entire health.

As promised I have provided you with, how to identify fructose, why it is bad for you and your family and how to eradicate it from your diet via my Fructose-Specific Food Charts.

*The Next Step is Yours!*

In this book I have touched on an Irritable Bowel Syndrome, Ileus, Blockage, Fibromyalgia, Adhesions, Narcotic Ileus, SIBO, Leaky Gut, Telescoping Intestines, Crohn's, Colitis, Celiac, Lactose, Sucrose, Uric Acid Levels and Gluten.

## Health Issues that have Similar or the Same Symptoms, have ONE ROOT PROBLEM—Diet

One thing they have all had in common is the negative impact of High Fructose Corn Syrup, as well as, similar symptoms, and how HFCS affects all of the illnesses listed.

Currently my concern is with our Medical Professionals… when did our Doctor's stop being Doctors?  When did they stop asking how and why we had an illness instead of just treating our symptoms?

Your, Doctors, Family and Friends may be throwing you a life raft in the form of prescription medications and surgeries, and you believe they are essential to fixing your problems.  You continue holding on as long as you can, waiting for the help that the drug companies and TV commercials promised you.  Only they don't deliver.  The truth is different…you possess the very power you need to improve your health.  You already have it, and you don't need prescriptions, treatments, or expensive experts to get it.

It is your ability to "Take" control of your life and become an educated patient as well as an educated consumer!

Keeping in mind how important our intestines are to our life remember they are similar to a root of a plant. Moreover, like roots our digestive tract absorbs nutrients from our food. Our intestinal wellbeing plays a vital place in whether we are well nourished.

I have provided you with supporting evidence of how HFCS decimates our health and in which areas of the body it takes place.

Your own incredible, body has the ability to recognize when something is not good for you. You need to listen…somewhere along the line (or at least the last 30– 35 years) we stopped listening to our body…we took the bait hook line and sinker.

We became complacent or lazy… we ate what we wanted, as often as we wanted and then we really screwed up our bodies by taking medication to fix the problem we just created. Our thought process was…I will just take a pill for it in the morning mentality and now that just doesn't fly!

It is amazing that for thousands of years the human body has been able to digest food choices with no problem…then over the last 35 years or so we have completely screwed our systems up with a barrage of multiple medications and synthetic foods and our bodies are telling us enough!

Stop and think about the marvel of the human body, that we don't have to tell ourselves to breathe… we breathe naturally; toxins are removed from our body by way of our liver and kidneys. The human body has always known how to "Detox" itself it hasn't stopped working…we have just given it more to deal with. What I'm sharing with you is not new information…perhaps temporarily misplaced but not new.

Depression, IBS, vitamin depletion, acidity, toxicity and serotonin productions all become lost pieces of a jig-saw puzzle that must connect on multiply levels in or to answer the how and why of our health.

*This is your turning point. All the symptoms you are experiencing may seem separate but they are linked by diet.*

In today's world, we have increased the level of toxins and have bombarded our systems with all types of synthetic food and additives and to what end?

We aren't any thinner, younger, or happier from these changes. We have developed more health issues in the last 30 years than we had 35 years ago.

There isn't one day that goes by without another pharmaceutical commercial encouraging us to be lazy and take their medication instead of eating properly.

I am not a doctor, I don't have a clinic, and I am not going provide you with a magic pill.

We have placed ourselves in a very precarious position by overloading our bodies with toxins. Our bodies are in a constant state of chronic inflammation and modern medicine knows that inflammation is the underlying cause for so many of health issues we face today.

We all have a boiling point...I've reached mine...when will you reach yours?

Eating healthy Organic food could prevent your blood pressure from rising or cause your cholesterol level to drop. Eating better improves the quality of your sleep, your level of energy and frame of mind.

I have provided you with all the information you need in this book to regain your digestive health. My question to you is...when will it be time for YOU to take back your life?

## Prior to Starting Your Fructose-Specific Food Charts:

If you have tested positive for any intolerance in addition to Fructose Intolerance such as...Celiac, Lactose, Gluten, SIBO, Leaky Gut or Irritable Bowel Syndrome you need to consider these health issues when planning your food selections. It will take a couple of weeks for your body to re-adjust.

To start I suggest you ask your doctor to order a blood panel. This will provide you with information in regards to any vitamin or mineral deficiencies.

Fructose Malabsorption, Leaky Gut, SIBO, and Irritable Bowel Syndrome will leave with some deficits in areas in which in turn can create a cascading effect on your health.

Discuss this with your doctor and move forward using the proper supplements but read the ingredients...fructose is in everything including medication. Be patient with your doctor...this is new territory for most of them.

To start:

1. Drink plenty of water and keep hydrated then wean yourself off juice, vitamin drinks, protein shakes, and flavored water. Read the labels this stuff has Fructose of some form in there ingredients. If you can't pronounce it, you shouldn't eat it.
2. Next, clean out your pantry and get rid of anything that has High Fructose Corn Syrup and Corn Syrup as part of the ingredients...all processed foods. Molasses and Honey are also a problem for Fructose challenged people. They have a naturally high level of Fructose and it's difficult for the body to break down.
3. Don't buy anything with "Fiber" added...this is inulin and is another word for Fructose. This is a synthetic ingredient. Get your fiber from natural foods.

4. Take your Fructose-Specific Food Charts with you or write down items from the charts that you want to eat. Buy fresh foods, nothing canned, frozen or pre-prepared. Organic is best but "Fresh" is a big step in the right direction.

5. All of the Fructose-Specific Foods are marked appropriately. Only consume 4 or 5 ounces of any item at one sitting. For example 5 ounces of chicken, 4 ounces of vegetable and 4 ounces of an approved fruit. As your brain re-trains your body, you can have larger portions.

6. Eat three meals a day and snacks in between. As long as you follow the Fructose-Specific Food Chart your body will be able to tolerate the selection...however, please keep in mind we all have different body chemistry. If you have a reaction to a food selection...take it off your list.

    a. After eating sit or lie down for approximately 15 minutes then get up and move around.
    b. You will find this helps with your blood sugar and with your digestion.
    c. If you lay on your right side after eating this can aid the stomach in emptying the contents to your small intestine.
    d. Eat small portions...stop eating before you feel uncomfortable.

7. Remember, natural and healthy are too different things so place a bookmark at these areas in your book for quick reference.

8. Plan your meals so you don't derail yourself. Fresh food is so much healthier for you...you will appreciate how good something tastes without the chemicals.

9. I have a page on Facebook, as well as a group, so I can assist you by providing you with the support of others. If you can't find a local support group, become part of mine.

10. I am a patient like you...I understand where you are coming from and where you want to go...only someone who has experienced the same issue can completely understand you and your needs.

11. Detox yourself without buying cleansing products. This can be done with selecting the correct foods and eating smaller than normal portions. This allows your body to have a rest...I have found after ingesting fructose that if I place myself on bowel rest for two days...I feel better much sooner. My personal bowel rest consists of drinking water and a small amount of protein once a day for the 2 – 3 days. This process keeps my Intestinal Tract in check.

12. Make sure you take some time to cogitate prior to setting your goals. Ultimately, your goal is to eat fresh and remove all processed food. Once you have done this, you will feel healthy again.

Your Expectations & Results

- I felt a bit overwhelmed and underprepared for my Fructose-Specific Food Life... but once I started to use my charts and took my appropriate supplements, it became very easy for me from that point on.
- I quit every beverage or food product that was even connected to *fructose* cold turkey.
- Within the first week, I started to feel better and the pain started to get bearable.
- By the end of week two, I noticed the bloating, gas and nausea was dissipating.
- After 30 days of eating my Fructose-Specific Foods, I had lost 25 pounds I stopped taking the medications, and never reached the level of intestinal debilitation again.
- After 65 days on my Fructose-Specific Food program, I had lost over 50 pounds. I realized my memory was much improved and nothing seemed as fuzzy as it once had.
- Six months after the initial start of eating Fructose-Specific foods, I found that my life was completely changed. I no longer was fatigued, angry, or achy.
- Many people believe that to empower one with the understanding of their own health is a life- altering event, it was for me, and I wanted to share that feeling with everyone!
- You will be amazed at how good you can feel.

At the most simplistic and literal level, "we are what we eat!" It is critical to understand how foods affect our bodies and know which foods to eliminate.

# Chapter Nineteen: What Your Eyes Say About Your Health

And the possible link between your Gut and Cholesterol Plaque. Many of you who have read my posts know I suffer from Hereditary Fructose Intolerance, as well as, other intolerances, fatigue etc. I had a TIA experience in August and was told all was well…this is a test you must have to verify that type of comment.

Can an eye exam save your life?

Things an Eye Doctor Can See

- Arterial plaques
- Hollenhorst plaques can be evidence of severe atherosclerosis. Ultrasound testing of the carotid arteries may be needed to pinpoint the plaque or plaques.
- Optic nerve abnormalities
- Retinal defects.

Ophthalmologists are always discussing the benefits of getting eyes examined regularly. Patients usually appreciate the importance of regular eye exams in detecting eye disease, but did you know that some conditions we look for can actually be life threatening?

One of those conditions can be revealed with an optomap Retinal exam. This is a laser scan for all comprehensive eye exam visits, to evaluate the health of the retina (the light sensitive tissue that lines the inside of the back of your eyes).

Why do we want to see the blood vessels?

Many disease states of the body can be revealed by analyzing the blood vessels for signs of a problem.

In this case, the patient has a blockage of one of the blood vessels in the retina (circled area in photo). Called a "retinal embolism" or Hollenhorst plaque, it's made up of cholesterol and came from a larger blood vessel elsewhere in the body.

Hollenhorst plaques found in the retina will prompt a phone call from our optometrist to your family doctor for special testing. The concern is that similar plaques could end up in the brain, causing a stroke or even death.

These plaques, if isolated to the retina, may or may not cause any symptoms whatsoever.

If small enough, the blood may work its way around them, but if slightly larger, the plaques may cause a loss of blood flow and even loss of vision.

Hollenhorst Plaque

Signs and Symptoms

The patient typically is elderly and often has concurrent history of hypertension, diabetes, carotid artery disease, peripheral vascular disease, hypercholesterolemia, hyperlipidemia, and/or atherosclerosis. The patient may be totally asymptomatic and the plaque(s) may be found on routine eye exam.

However, the patient may have previously experienced transient episodes of monocular blindness (amaurosis fugax). Rarely, the patient has experienced a transient ischemic attack with hemiparesis, paraesthesia, and/or aphasia.

These episodic bouts of amaurosis fugax may be quite frequent, and may last from several seconds to several minutes. Rarely does the patient have any lasting visual deficits.

Frequently, the patient previously experiencing amaurosis fugax will not exhibit retinal emboli, but may have arteriolar narrowing and sheathing. A Hollenhorst plaque appears as a bright, glistening, refractile plaque, usually at the bifurcation of a retinal arteriole. These have the propensity to break up and move, and may not be present at subsequent visits.

The association between Retinal cholesterol emboli (RCE, "Hollenhorst plaques") RCE and cardiovascular disease has been recognized since Hollenhorst's original paper on the eponymous plaques in 1961.

Subsequent clinical questions addressed the relationship between the presence of RCE and the risk of associated mortality from vascular occlusive disease, but recent studies have focused on medical work-up after discovery of RCE.

One critically important distinction that has emerged from this corpus is an assessment of RCE within the context of patient visual symptomatology.

## HOW FOOD ADDITIVES TIE INTO THE INCREASE OF HOLLENHORST PLAQUE

Recently, I have read several articles written my Ophthalmologists and this is their take on how our processed food affects our body— specifically our eyes. I do not have peer review research but I believe the information I have shared is something you could ask your doctor about and check to see what you might find on published articles for this issue.

To read an article in its entirety please go to:
http://lowcarboptometrist.blogspot.com/

The three paragraphs below came from the article attached to the site I just provided to you.

Many Ophthalmologists, more and more each year, evidence of cholesterol in the eyes of patients has increased. Indeed, even if there truly is more cholesterol seen nowadays in peoples' eyes (i.e., five years ago an eye doctor would see only 1 patient a day with cholesterol in their eyes, now they would see 3-5 patients a day with cholesterol in their eyes), what would that mean? What would it matter? Sure, if an embolism is present in a retinal artery, this can have a disastrous effect on ocular health and vision. But, if cholesterol is building up in the cornea (arcus), does it mean anything? Does it matter?

Lastly, one more group of related questions- and this is probably where I'm trying to go- do I believe in the cholesterol-heart disease hypothesis or the lipid hypothesis? Do I follow along with the health, food and political industries (among others, these last few decades) that say we all need to eat low fat, high-carb diets to keep heart-healthy?

Do I really agree with these same industries that say we are fat or obese because we are lazy (don't exercise enough) and we have no self-control (eat too much)? Is "a calorie a calorie" and is saturated fat to blame for everything un-"healthy"?

Well, I think there are many more questions to ask (and much deeper ones as well) but let's start there.

Maybe the health care field is too busy to talk about eating REAL FOOD while cutting down on or eliminating processed foods and sugars...too busy to discuss the possibility that maybe what we feed our bodies-what we eat- does have a tremendous affect on our health. Let's continue the discussion and continue asking questions, until we can find the underlying cause of the food we eat and the impact on the entire body.

If you have cholesterol embolization and it is partially blocking small to medium arteries and affecting nerves to the gut…the blood flow will decrease and impact the health of that particular digestive organ "could be" affected.

Cholesterol embolization syndrome refers to embolization of the contents of an atherosclerotic plaque (primarily cholesterol crystals) from a proximal large-caliber artery to distal small to medium arteries causing end-organ damage by mechanical plugging and an inflammatory response. Synonyms used in the medical literature include atheromatous embolization, cholesterol crystal embolization, and atheroembolism.

The gastrointestinal symptoms have been described in 18.6 - 48% of cholesterol embolization syndromes. Gut ischaemia is the primary mode of presentation with associated intestinal blood loss. The symptoms include abdominal pain nausea and vomiting.

Blood loss is typically chronic with bleeding occurs from mucosal ulcerations or infarcts. These lesions are microscopic and are easily missed in endoscopy and other radiological studies.

If emboli (Emboli: Something that travels through the bloodstream, lodges in a blood vessel and blocks it. Examples of emboli are a detached blood clot, a clump of bacteria, and foreign materials). (Cholesterol embolism/Hollenhorst Plaques) have spread to the digestive tract, reduced appetite, nausea and vomiting may occur, as well as nonspecific abdominal pain, gastrointestinal hemorrhage (vomiting blood, or admixture of blood in the stool), and occasionally acute pancreatitis (inflammation of the pancreas).

Renal atheroembolism can lead to acute, sub-acute, and chronic renal failure. In acute and subacute forms, an inciting event can be elicited. In contrast, chronic forms are likely due to spontaneous low-grade release of cholesterol emboli over long periods. The prognosis of atheroembolic renal disease is considered to be poor with reported mortality varying from 70 to 90%.

Kidney involvement leads to the symptoms of renal failure, which are non-specific but usually cause nausea, reduced appetite (anorexia) , raised blood pressure (hypertension), and occasionally the various symptoms of electrolyte disturbance such as an irregular heartbeat. Some patients report hematuria (bloody urine) but this may only be detectable on microscopic examination of the urine.

Increased amounts of protein in the urine may cause edema (swelling) of the skin (a combination of symptoms known as nephrotic syndrome).

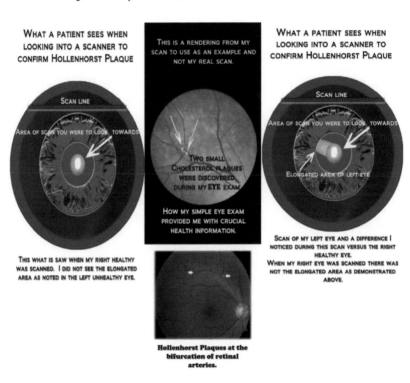

WHAT A PATIENT SEES WHEN LOOKING INTO A SCANNER TO CONFIRM HOLLENHORST PLAQUE

THIS IS A RENDERING FROM MY SCAN TO USE AS AN EXAMPLE AND NOT MY REAL SCAN.

WHAT A PATIENT SEES WHEN LOOKING INTO A SCANNER TO CONFIRM HOLLENHORST PLAQUE

SCAN LINE

AREA OF SCAN YOU WERE TO LOOK TOWARDS

TWO SMALL CHOLESTEROL PLAQUES WERE DISCOVERED DURING MY EYE EXAM

SCAN LINE

AREA OF SCAN YOU WERE TO LOOK TOWARDS

ELONGATED AREA OF LEFT EYE

HOW MY SIMPLE EYE EXAM PROVIDED ME WITH CRUCIAL HEALTH INFORMATION.

THIS WHAT IS SAW WHEN MY RIGHT HEALTHY WAS SCANNED. I DID NOT SEE THE ELONGATED AREA AS NOTED IN THE LEFT UNHEALTHY EYE.

SCAN OF MY LEFT EYE AND A DIFFERENCE I NOTICED DURING THIS SCAN VERSUS THE RIGHT HEALTHY EYE.
WHEN MY RIGHT EYE WAS SCANNED THERE WAS NOT THE ELONGATED AREA AS DEMONSTRATED ABOVE.

Hollenhorst Plaques at the bifurcation of retinal arteries.

297

TIPS FOR SHOPPING, BAKING, AND COOKING WITH HFI

# Publix Markets 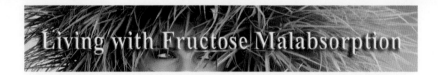 Fresh Market

Whole Foods carry a "Cola" that is all natural but it is not for Diabetics due to the fact it is Sweetened by sugar.

Look for an Organic grocery store. I love to shop at Whole Foods and Publix but if you don't have either in your town look for the organic section in your own grocery store.

I strongly suggest giving up all carbonated beverages, as it will improve your digestive tract.

My suggestions are based on my Hereditary Fructose Intolerance and is not meant to cover every intolerance. Please keep that in mind!

I am in the processing of creating a cookbook that will encompass all of the Food Intolerances and the needs of those individuals.

Interesting Note: Sweet Tarts are almost pure glucose (on the label, you will see Dextrose as the ingredient) and so someone with HFI or FM this can be tolerated and considered medicine of sorts.

It is likely that for some reason you will not be able to maintain your Fructose diet or you're going to eat something that you probably shouldn't have if that happens… take a Sweet tarts about 5-10 minutes prior to ingesting the non-tolerated food.

This will give your system extra glucose to process the incoming fructose. Sweet-Tarts are made up of Dextrose, which is a powered Glucose.

This will only work for excess fructose but not fructans (wheat and onions) -although this helps, it is not a cure.

The body still has a total fructose tolerance level and no matter how much glucose you consume, it's going to suffer if you eat too much fructose.

This will only work if they are the original Sweet tarts. The label will mention Dextrose as the main ingredient.

For those die-hard cola drinkers I have this tip to offer you! One quick tip...if you are going to die without drinking a cola...make sure it is worth the pain and make sure it is imported from Mexico.

Yes, I said .Mexico; because Mexico uses real sugar to sweeten their drinks...we (The United States) use HFCS to sweeten our sodas, as well as, vitamin water and much, much more!

Don't you think it is strange that we have to import a Cola from Mexico in order to have the original ingredients from a soft drink that was made in this country? Mexico will not sell our Cola due to the fact it is Sweetened by HFCS or Corn Syrup.

This is not Gluten Free but if you can tolerate rye flour I use it for my pie crusts.

# NOTE: I am working on a cookbook to make and bake life easier.

Pie Crusts: This can be tricky I use a regular piecrust recipe but I add 1/8 cup of dextrose to the flour prior to adding the butter to flour. This gives me a slight advantage for the Fructose-Glucose ratio and swings the balance to my favor...so now the crust will have a higher Glucose ratio and your small intestines can break it down.

This may not work for everyone but it has worked for me! Also, note, I use organic butter.

Fillings: I can make the following pies, fresh strawberry, fresh blueberry, fresh raspberry, Pumpkin and Lemon Meringue. When creating a filling for your piecrust you must use fresh fruit and replace the amount of sugar with a sugar substitute you can tolerate. I use Stevia and my berry pies turn out great.

Always use as much organic products as possible. I know it is expensive to make a berry pie because you are paying for fresh fruit not a canned product.

Pumpkin Pie filling can be tolerated even in a can if it is pure pumpkin.

Look on the label to make sure it is pure pumpkin and not a prepared pumpkin filling. If you use the pure pumpkin with condensed milk (not canned sweetened milk...there is a difference) substitute the amount of sugar with Stevia or the sugar substitute you have found effective (don't use any sugar substitute that is listed on the "DON'T" list...for Fructose Malabsorption or HFI.

If you don't use the proper substitute, you will not be able to reduce your intestinal issues or enjoy this pie!

Lemon Meringue...this is in a box but is made from dextrose, which can be broken down properly in your system. When making the Meringue use your sugar substitute and brown as you usually would.

The only pies I can eat...are the ones I can make from scratch and the ingredients must be fresh and natural. I can enjoy the following: Blueberry, Raspberry, Strawberry, Pumpkin, and Lemon.

Homemade Whipped Cream: (Obviously, not for lactose intolerant individuals) Use organic heavy whipping cream one pint. Make homemade powder sugar. This consists of one cup of raw sugar crystals 1/4 cup of dextrose and two cups of Stevia.

Place the ingredients into a blender until you have a very fine powder and you know all three ingredients are mixed well....this will be more than needed for just one batch of whipped cream so keep the fine powder in a sealed container.

Once the whipped cream is made, it lasts for approximately 3 days in the fridge.

Jams: As you know making any kind of Jam, Jelly, or Syrup takes a tremendous amount of sugar. You can now enjoy these treats by substituting your sugar your tolerated sweetener.

Once again you must use fresh ingredients...it is not cheap but it is healthy and your system will be able to process this food selection. I use organic fruit and I don't use pectin.

I had never canned before in my life but I soon found myself buying the items that were necessary to can...and in turn, the process provides me with a chance to enjoy Jams and Jelly. I wouldn't have been able to digest these items if I had not made them from scratch.

Sandwiches: Use wraps when you want a sandwich. I have only found one kind of bread that I can tolerate it is Rye bread from rye flour...it is listed under a "Maybe able to Tolerate" item but for 18 months I have been able to eat one piece a day without repercussions.

I have had to roast my own beef and turkey since processed food has too many unknowns...but I have found buy roasting my own meats and slicing them, I am sure of what I am getting.

I store the pre-cooked meats in baggies and store them in packages in my fridge. This provides me with a quick fix or a lunch to go!

Spaghetti Sauce: I don't recommend this very often but when you just have to have it follow these directions for the least amount of repercussions.

Use organic tomato paste...do not use canned tomato sauce...you can use the paste and mix it with three cans of water to each can of paste. You can cut up shallots, use fresh sweet basil, fresh oregano, fresh rosemary, olive oil, and garlic water.  I also use one-fourth cup of dextrose to increase the glucose from the paste.

For garlic water take a cup of water and place 2 or 3 cloves of garlic (peeled) in the cup and put in the microwave on high or boil water on the stove and pour the boiling water into the cup that has the garlic...either way is fine.

Let the cloves of garlic steep in the hot water for 20 minutes and then when you are making your sauce use the garlic water for the flavor. You get the taste but not the garlic that you can't digest.

Ketchup::  I but organic ketchup...read the label and make sure you know what is in the ketchup it can be organic and still have Agave as a sweetener!  Agave is not good for you!

 I take organic ketchup open it up and add 1 teaspoon of dextrose to the pre-made ketchup...once again it changes the fructose-glucose ratio to my favor and I can digest it without problems. Don't abuse!

Munchies:   We all love them but now you have to be more selective...there are a couple types of organic chips on the market that you can enjoy...but don't overload your system with these products an overabundance can create problems.   There are all natural potato chips and they can be found in your organic section of your grocery store. Make sure you are getting the plain type of chips. Flavored chips will hurt you!

I have found one brand of corn chips that I can eat.  Read the labels carefully, the ingredients must be all natural...that someone with HFI or FM can digest.

Now, here is a tip...you can buy salsa separate the actual pieces of veggies out of it and use the juice that is left as your dip.
 It is the pieces of veggies your body can't digest you can still enjoy the flavor as long as you follow this process...only eat on occasion.

Eating Out: in all honesty, this is not easy! Eating out is not just about the food you eat…it is a huge portion of how we interact with friends and work associates.

A couple of restaurants would be Chipotle's and Zoe's Kitchen.

Eating out is "Synonymous" with how we socialize. Our lives revolve around food. We use it to celebrate, as well as, mourn. We spend the majority of our time with family and friends…eating and drinking.

You can order a baked potato, romaine lettuce salad and some shellfish I suggest if you order crab legs that you bring your own organic butter and request that they melt it for you…many restaurants use more of a butter oil and not real butter.

A glass of white wine…Sauvignon Blanc…I have found this to be the driest white wine for my system and I will have 4 ounces without any problems.

You need to take in account that each winery and the location of the winery can have varying levels of what is considered "Dry" wine. Find one that you can tolerate and stick to that brand.

The three images of me pictured below demonstrate what removing Fructose from my diet did for my health. In March of 2013, I started exercising again to regain my strength and endurance.

If you look at my face in the picture on the left below, you can see it is no longer swollen or puffy and the image on the right demonstrates how much weight I lost after removing as much *fructose* as possible.

## I'm feeling "Healthier & Happier!"

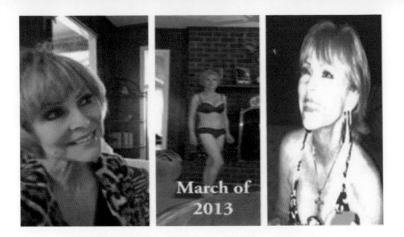

They say a picture is worth a thousand words!

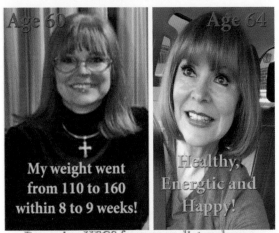

My weight went from 110 to 160 within 8 to 9 weeks!

Healthy, Energtic and Happy!

Removing HFCS from your diet makes an incredible difference in your life!

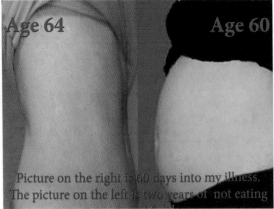

Picture on the right is 60 days into my illness. The picture on the left is two years of not eating

My food choices were not made because of my weight...they were made because of my health and the poor quality of life I was experiencing. This is not an example of an <u>image issue or self-esteem problem</u> this is what processed foods did to me!

Removing Fructose provided me with the added benefit of getting back to a healthier weight. Organic, real food is the only way I can survive. No more fast food canned or pre-packaged for me!

I eat frequently, I eat fresh, and I eat ORGANIC!

## I leave you with this...

High-fructose corn syrup (HFCS) is a liquid sweetener alternative to sucrose (table sugar) used in most foods and beverages. Early developmental work was carried out in the 1960's, with shipments of the first commercial HFCS product to the food industry occurring in the late 1960's. Phenomenal growth over the ensuing 35 or more years made <u>HFCS one of the most successful food ingredients in modern history</u>.

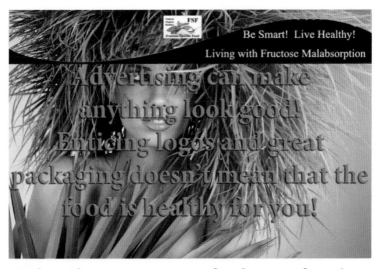

## What do you want to feed your family?

# Special and Sincere Thanks!

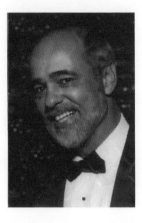

I want to thank my husband <u>Paul,</u> who went through as much hell as I did and yet stayed with me. It was not an easy task for anyone. If you are in constant pain...you are not a nice person. He not only had the frustration of not knowing how to help me...he also went through every day of pain with me. He never thought I had a drug problem or that it was in my head and I thank him for that. He just wanted me to get help and feel better...Thanks Paul...I love you!

I want to thank all of my children but an extra thanks to my <u>son Ed, his wife Jennifer of Boston and my daughter Jessica and her husband Greg of Charlotte, my friends Karen McBride and Dr. Luke Curtsinger of Savannah, Georgia</u> for encouraging me to write this book. Friends are blessings. In closing, I want to acknowledge my doctor's who "WERE" helpful during this process.

I had mentioned early on that I had experienced a horrible situation with an ER Doctor at the hospital I go to in I frequented. After being diagnosed, I requested a meeting with him. It took 16 months but he did sit down with me, he looked at my information, and promised me he would think about this situation as a possible solution to his future ER patients. I only had one reason for meeting with him. I thought it was extremely important that he too, was educated on health issue of *Fructose.*

Disclaimer: The information and advice presented are no way intended to be a substitute for medical counseling. This book was created for you to share with your physician. Please make sure you consult your physician before changing your lifestyle as I have. You and I are both human but we each have unique body chemistry and this differs from person to person.

The information in this book is based on my research of over 3,000 pages of documentation that I have condensed down for the first time. The research was created after months of tedious hours of reading articles, medical journals, library, and medical research resources that I could share when writing my personal story. It was because of my severe health issues and months of reading and researching that I can now spare you the time and spread the word of Hereditary Fructose Intolerance and Fructose Malabsorption.

I am providing the information in one spot in order to help you feel better!

The advice presented is in no way intended to be a substitute for medical counseling.

I am not a Doctor, Nurse nor am I a dietician...but I am a patient with this problem. For over 2 1/2 years, I had no help. The endless hours in the ER and hospital admissions, the outpatient tests, scans, blood work, MRI's, as well as, the hundreds of hours of reading and research in regards to this Journey provided me with the credentials to discuss this health issue with you.

MY CONTACT INFORMATION IS:

Feel free to email me at  IBShelpishere@comcast.net

My website is  www.IBSHelpishere.net

Facebook: https://.facebook.com/IBSHelpisHere

## Be Smart! Live Healthy!

# NOOK REVIEWS:

**Reader -** *Karen McBride*
Karen found this book is easy to understand and read for both the patient and the professional.

**Reader –** *Joy Hill*
Joy found the book to be a wealth of information and loved the fact that actual food charts were included. Now she knows what she can and can't eat.

**Reader –** *Carol Danilak*
I found the charts to be very user friendly and I started feeling better within weeks.

**Reader –***Karen Staggs*
I was surprised that eating as suggested could bring on such quick results. I lost 15 pounds in 35 days.

## Be Smart! Live Healthy!

1. http://medicine.med.nyu.edu/conditions-we-treat/conditions/ileus#sthash.iXJNBV3d.dpuf, See more at:. *Diagnosis Ileus.* Savannah : Nancie Paruso, 2012. 1.

2. Bowel Blockage Merriam-Webster's Medical Dictionary, Barrons Medical Guides Dictionary of Medical Terms, Gray's Anatomy, Guide to Pathology, Forensic Science and Investigator and Handbook, s. General Research. *Bowel Blockage.* p. 21.

3. Paruso, Nancie. *Diagnosis Fibromyalgia.* 2012.

4. Adhesions from Archive Files of Harvard Medical, Mayo Clinic and Boston University. *Diagnosis Adhesions.* 2012. p. 22.

5. SIBO, Merriam Webster's Medical Dictionary, Barron's Dictionary of Medical Terms, Guide to Pathology, Forensic Science, Archives of Harvard Medical, Boston University, Mayo Clinic and University of Iowas. SIBO Small Intestine Bacterial Overgrowth. pp. 27-28.

6. Siebecker, Dr. Allison. p. 28.

7. —. *Quote.* 2012.

8. 27-Nov-2012, Public release date:. Hiagh Fructose Corn Syrup Global Prevalence of Diabetes Link!

9. Paruso, Nancie. *Diagnosis Leaky Gut.* 2012.

10. Colitis and Crohn's Disease Merriam Webster's Medical Dictionary, Barron's Dictionary of Medical Terms, Archives of Harvard Medical, University of Iowa, Boston University and Mayo Clinic. Diagnosis Ulcerative Colitis and Crohn's Disease. 2012, pp. 29-30.

11. Research, Compiled. *Diagnosis Irritabel Bowel Disease.* 2012.

12. Page 1. Ciccone A, Allegra JR, Cochrane DG, Cody RP, Roche LM. Age-related differences in diagnoses within the elderly population. Am J Emerg Med 1998 and 16:43-48. Unrelenting Pain.

13. Chronic Pain Fact Sheet/by Marcia E. Bedard, PhD.

14. 1 American Chronic Pain Association. "Coping with Chronic Pain." 1995, Brownlee, Shannon, and Joannie M. Schrof. "The Quality of Mercy." U.S. News and World Report, 2 March 17, 1997: 55-57, 60-62, 65, 67, 3 Pasero, Christine L., R.N., B.S.N., and Margo M. Chronic Pain Fact Sheet/by Marcia E. Bedard, PhD.

15. HFCS Introduction. Abstract/FREE Full Text Salomonsson I. Shelf life: sucrose hydrolysis. Copenhagen, Denmark: Danisco Sugar A/S, 2005. Internet: www.danisco.com/cms/resources/file/eb241b041a6ed65/Shelf%2 0life.pdf (accessed 15 March 2007). When was High Fructose Corn Syrup Introduced. 2012, p. 57.

16. *Diagnosis Hereditary Fructose Intolerance.* Hereditary Fructose Intolerance, HFI Laboratory at Boston University: Specifics of HFI and Its. 2012, pp. 41-44.

17. Syrup, What is High Fructose Corn, Jump up ^ Agriculture and Agri-Food Canada: The Canadian Soft Drink Industry "Glucose/fructose is a generic term for high fructose corn syArchives of Harvard Medical, Boston University, University of Iowa and Mayo Clinic. What is High Fructose Corn Syrup. 2012, pp. 54-55.

18. Referenced: 21 ^ Marshall, R. O., Kooi, E. R. and Moffett, G. M. (1957). "Enzymatic Conversion of d-Glucose to d-Fructose".

Science 125 (3249): 648–649. doi:10.1126/science.125.3249.648. PMID 13421660. edit 22 Jump up ^ Yamanaka K (1966). "[104] d-Xylose. How is HFCS Produced? 2012, p. 55.

19. Research. *Fructose Absorption by the Body.* 2012 .

20. Fructose, First Affects of. How Does HFCS First Affect the Human Body? 2012, pp. 64-65.

21. Six, http://www.ibshelpishere.net/contents.html see-- Chapter.

22. http://www.sciencedaily.com/releases/1998/11/981126103305.ht m. Story Source: The above story is based on materials provided by American Technion Society.Note: Materials may be edited for content and length. *1998.*

23. William Misner, PhD. Fructose Increases the Rate of Aging.

24. http://www.eidon.com/diabetes2.htmol. Eidon Diabetes . *2002.*

25. Mercola, Dr. If you want to age gracefully! *http://www.huffingtonpost.com/dr-mercola/if-you-want-to-age-gracef_b_700335.html.* 2010.

26. Depression, Merriam-Webster's Medical Dictionary, Barron's Dictionary of Medical Terms, Gray's Anatomy, Guide to Pathology, Archieved files from Harvard Medical, Boston University, University of Iowa and Mayo Clinic. Depression & Depleted Vitamins and Minerals. 2012, pp. 72-76.

27. Uric Acid Levels, Merriam-Webster's Medical Dictionary, Barron's Dictionary of Medical Terms, Guide to Pathology, Gray's Anatomy, Archives from Harvard Medical, Boston

University, Mayo Clinic and University of Iowa. Uric Acid Levels as Marker for Fructose. pp. 75-76.

28. AGE Advanced Glycation End, Barron's Dictionary of Medical Terms, Gray's Anatomy, Guide to Pathology, Archives Files from Harvard Medical, Boston University and University of Iowa. AGE Advanced Glycation End. pp. 77-78.

29. *5 Reason High Fructose Corn Syrup will kill you!* References:: Dufault, R., LeBlanc, B., Schnoll, R. et al. 2009. Mercury from chlor-alkali plants: Measured concentrations in food product sugar. Environ Health. 26(8):2. (ii) Bray, G.A., Nielsen, S.J., and B.M. Popkin. 2004. Consumption of high-fructose. 2011, pp. 86-92.

30. Ernst J. Schaefer 1-3, 4,* Joi A. Gleason, 4 and Michael L. Dansinger5. *Dietary Fructose and Glucose Differentially Affect Lipid and Glucose Homeostasis.* 2012.

31. Mark Hyman, MD. High Fructose Corn Syrup. *2012.*

32. American, Reference: By Adam Hadhazy Scientific. Think Twice - How the Gut's "Second Brain" Influces Mood and Well Being. 2012, pp. 101-103.

33. Reference: Autism Speaks November 13, 2013. *Autism Speaks.* 2013. pp. 101-103.

34. Alzheimer's. Statisics. 2013.

35. Prebiotics, Barron's dictionary of Medical terms, Gray's Anatomy & Merriam-Webster Medical Dictionary. Prebiotics and Probiotics. pp. 117-119.

36. Georgia, Dr Rao of Augusta.

37. Medicine, Keck School of. University of Southern California's Keck School of Medicine. 2012, pp. 129-131.

38. medicine, Arizona advanced. *http://arizonaadvancedmedicine.com/autoimmune-diseases/*.

39. Paruso, Nancie. *Fructose Research.* Savannah : s.n., 2012.

40. 1, High Fructose Corn Syrup and interesting ways to create pandemics. Part. Ralph Turchiano. *Http://healthresearchreport.me/2013/12/04/high-fructose-corn-syrup-interesting-ways-to-create-pandemics-part-1/.* 2013.

41. Kim Irwin All Posts, Consumer Products, Sweetners • Tags: American Journal of Clinical Nutrition, HFCS, High-fructose corn syrup, Jonsson Comprehensive Cancer Center, National Institutes of Health, Sugar, U.S. News & World Report, United States. pancreatic cancers use high fructose corn syrup (HFCS), common in the Western diet to fuel their growth. *American Journal of Clinical Nutrition.* University of California Los Angeles, Vol. kirwin@mednet.ucla.edu.

42. Blaise W. LeBlanc, Ph.D. Carl Hayden Bee Research Center http://pubs.acs.org/stoken/presspac/presspac/full/10.1021/jf901 4526. *Research Center Agricultural Research Service U.S. Department of Agriculture Tucson AZ.* General Diet, Other Food Additives, Sweetners Tags: Agricultural Research Service, Colony collapse disorder, HFCS, High-fructose corn syrup, HMF, Honey bee, Hydroxymethylfurfural, Journal of Agricultural and Food Chemistry, United States .

43. California, Leslie Ridgeway Univeristy of Southern. High Fructose Corn Syrup Global Prevalence of Diabetes Link! *University of Southern California.* 2012 November 27th.

44. (2012), Goran M Ulijaszek S. and Ventura E. High Fructose corn syrup and diabestes prevlance: A global perspective. *Global Public Health.* 2012, November 27.

45. Aoki, Gary Taubes and Kenji. New York Times 2009 Article on Robert Lustig. *Is Sugar Toxic.* Ralph Finennes, 2011 April 13, Vols. • Sweet and Vicious (May 1, 2011) .

46. Parsuo, Nancie. *Diagnosis Narcotic Ileus.* 2012.

47. Paruso, Nancie. *Diagnosis SIBO.* 2012.

48. Research, Compiled. *Diagnosis Hereditary Fructose Intolerance.* 2012.

49. Medical, Harvard. *Brain Gut Connection.* 2012.

50. Ileus, Merriam Webster's Medical Dictionary, Grays Anatomy, Baroons Dictional of Medical Tersm, Guide to Pathology and Forensic Science. *2010-2012.* Page 17.

51. Fibromyalgia Merriam Webster's Medical Dicationary, Guide to Pathology, Gray's Anantomy, Barrons Dictionaly of Medical Terms, Archive files from Harvard and Boston College. p. 21.

52. Narcotic Ileus Merriam Webster's Medical Dictionary, Gray's Anatomy , Guide to Pathology , Barrons Dictionary of Medical Terms, Archives from Harvard Medical, University of Iowa, Boston University and Mayo Clinic. Narcotic Ileus. p. 22.

53. Telescoping Intestine Merriam Webster's Medical Dictionary, Barron's Dictionary of Medical Terms, Gray's Anatomy, Gude to Pathology and Forensic Science. Diagnosis Telecoping Intestine. pp. 28-29.

54. Syndrome, Irritable Bowel and Merriam Webster's Medical Dictionary, Barron's Dictionary of Medical Terms, Gray's Anatomy, Guide to Pathology Forensic Science, Archives from Harvard Medical University, University of Iowa, Boston University and Mayo Clinic. *Diagnosis Irritabel Bowel Disease.* 2012. pp. 34-35.

55. What is Fructose, Merriam-Webster's Medical Dictionary, Barron's Dictionary of Medical Terms, Archived Files, Harvard Medical. Fructose. p. 38.

56. Sources:http://www.seedsofdeception.com/Public/AboutGenetic allyModifiedFoods/index.cfm. Six Negative Facts. pp. 179-180.

57. Brain Gut Connection, Archieve Files from Harvard Medical, Boston UniversityBy Barbara Bradley Bolen, Ph.D, About.com Guide. Gut Brain Connection. 2012, pp. 97-100.

58. Clinic, Mayo. *Diagnosis Adhesions.* 2012.

59. *What is High Fructose Corn Syrup.* 2012.

60. Diagnosis, HFI Laboratory at Boston University: Specifics of HFI and Its. *Diagnosis Hereditary Fructose Intolerance.* 2012.

61. http://www.ncbi.nlm.nih.gov/pmc/articles/PMC3378453/, Source.

62. Froelich, Amanda. Are you Consuming the 9 most genetically modified foods? *Knowledge is Truth.* March 2014.

63. Hopkins, Johns. Years of telling people chemotheragpy is the only way to try (Try, being the key word) to eliminate cancer. Johns Hopkins is finally starting to tell you there is an alternative way. *Johns Hopkins Cancer Update.* 2014.

64. McAuliff, Michael. Huffington Post. *FOLLOW: Bernie Sanders, Video, GMO Labeling, GMO Labeling Senate, Senate GMOs, Bernie Sanders Gmo, Bernie Sanders Gmos, Fda, Genetically Modified Food, Genetically Modified Organisms, Gmo, Gmo Food, Gmo Labeling Bill, Gmo News, monsanto, Monsanto Gmos, St.*

65. William Misner, PhD. Fructose Increases the Rate of Aging . *2002.*

66. Mercola, Dr. Fructose and Alzheimer's Disease. *Category Archieves Alzheimer's Disease.* Dr. Mercola article from 2012 on Alzheimer's , 2012, pp. 104-107.

67. 1. http://medicine.med.nyu.edu/conditions-we-treat/conditions/ileus#sthash.iXJNBV3d.dpuf, See more at:. Diagnosis Ileus. Savannah : Nancie Paruso, 2012. 1.

68. Marcia E. Bedard, PhD. Chronic Pain Fact Shee.

69. 308, Multiple see 307 to. The "Negative" Impact of Unrelenting Pain.

70. Page 1. Ciccone A, Allegra JR, Cochrane DG, Cody RP, Roche LM. Age-related differences in diagnoses within the elderly population. Am J Emerg Med 1998 and 16:43-48. Under Treatment of Acute Pain.

71. PHD, Marcia Bedard. Chronic Pain Fact Sheet.

## SIBO - In-depth

In plain terms is an overgrowth of bacteria in your small intestines.

It is a common of IBS and digestive problems like bloating, gas, abdominal pain, diarrhea, and constipation by fermenting any types of carbohydrates you eat (starches and sugars).

In addition, SIBO is often associated with a leaky gut. If your gut is leaky, it will let large undigested food particles in your bloodstream, causing systemic symptoms such as skin rash, headaches, joint pain, autoimmune disorders, etc. Leaky gut is a common cause of food intolerances.

Correcting the bacterial overgrowth and healing & sealing your leaky gut should help you feel a lot better.

Specific antibiotics or herbal antibiotics (under a naturopathic doctor's supervision) can be used to speed up the treatment of SIBO.

Small intestinal bacterial overgrowth (SIBO), also termed bacterial overgrowth, or Small bowel bacterial overgrowth syndrome (SBBOS), is a disorder of excessive bacterial growth in the small intestine. Unlike the colon (or large bowel), which is rich with bacteria, the small bowel usually has fewer than 10 organisms per milliliter. Patients with bacterial overgrowth typically develop symptoms including nausea, bloating, vomiting, diarrhea, malnutrition, weight loss, and malabsorption, which are caused by a number of mechanisms.

The diagnosis of bacterial overgrowth is made by a number of techniques, with the gold standard diagnosis being an aspirate from the jejunum that grows in excess of 10 bacteria per millilitre.

Small bowel bacterial overgrowth syndrome is treated with antibiotics, which may be given in a cyclic fashion to prevent tolerance to the antibiotics.

Risk factors for the development of bacterial overgrowth include the use of medications, possibly including proton pump inhibitors, anatomical disturbances in the bowel, including fistulae, diverticulitis, and blind loops created after surgery, and resection of the ileo-cecal valve.

(7) Dr. Allison Siebecker states: Dr. Siebecker

The main symptoms of SIBO are those of Irritable Bowel Syndrome (IBS). SIBO has been shown to exist in up to 84% of IBS patients (but those patients were not tested for Fructose Malabsorption. Therefore, SIBO is theorized to be the underlying cause. It is associated with many other disorders, as well as, an underlying cause or after effect of the pre-existing disease.

In particular, if the symptoms of IBS are present, or one of the associated diseases along with digestive symptoms is present, consider SIBO.

According to Bures et al, "It is mandatory to consider SIBO in all cases of complex non-specific dyspeptic complaints (bloating, abdominal discomfort, diarrhea, abdominal pain), in motility disorders, anatomical abnormalities of the small bowel and in all malassimilation syndromes (malabsorption, maldigestion).

Associated Conditions- see SIBO Diseases for Study links  Associated issues below:      Acne Roseacea, Acromegaly, Age: Elderly, Alcohol Consumption (moderate intake), Anemia, Autism, Celiac Disease, Chronic Fatigue Syndrome, CLL (Chronic Lymphocytic Leukemia), Cystic Fibrosis, Diabetes, Diverticulitis, Dyspepsi, Erosive Esophagitis, Fibromyalgia, Gallstones, Gastroparesis, GERD (Gastroesophageal Reflux Disease), Hepatic Encephalopathy (Minimal) H pylori Infection, Hyprochlorhydria, Hypothyroid/ Hashimoto's Thyroiditis, IBD (Inflammatory Bowel Disease), -Crohn's, -Ulcerative Colitis, IBS (Irritable Bowel Syndrome), Interstitial Cystitis, L, Lactose Intolerance, Liver cirrhosis, Lyme, Medications: Proton Pump Inhibitors, Opiates, Muscular Dystrophy (myotonic Type 1), NASH/NAFLD (non-alcoholic: steatohepatitis/fatty liver disease), Obesity, Pancreatitis, Parasites, Parkinson's, Prostatitis (chronic), Restless Leg Syndrome, Rheumatoid Arthritis, Scleroderma

Surgery: Post-Gastrecomy

For more details, see an article called:

SIBO: Often Ignored Cause of IBS by Dr. Allison Siebecker

"My mission is to share information and news about SIBO

To empower people in their health." Dr. Allison Siebecker

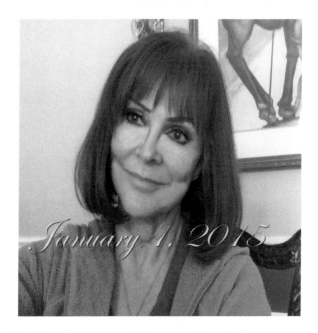

Eating Healthy, Removing all Processed Foods from your diet can
and will make a difference!

Good Health to all!\\

This condition occurs due to gaps in the membrane lining of your intestinal tract. These tiny gaps allow toxic substance that should be confined to your digestive tract to escape into your bloodstream – hence the term leaky gut syndrome. Leaky Gut can cause you to pack on the pounds and it demonstrates very similar symptoms.

With leaky gut, not only is the digestive lining more porous and less selective about what can get in, but normal absorption can also be affected.

Nutritional deficiencies may develop because of damage to the villi – the finger-like projections in the small intestine that are responsible for absorbing nutrients.

Possible Symptoms are as follows:

Disrupt the small intestine, Bloating, Pain, Unexplained ailments of the intestine

Our small intestine, which is responsible for about 70% of our immune system, behaves like a selective sieve: it lets only nutrients and well-digested fats, proteins, and starches enter the bloodstream and keeps out large molecules, microbes, and toxins.

Leaky gut syndrome happens when the intestinal lining becomes inflamed, and the microvilli on the lining become damaged; this prevents the microvilli from absorbing nutrients and producing necessary enzymes and secretions for healthy digestion and absorption.

Two things were certain:

- The Gut- Brain connection is clear
- Leaky Gut Syndrome is exacerbated this food additive

Our current lifestyle that includes diets high in this substance can bring an enormous amount of pain and frustration to those who suffer from leaky gut. Klebsiella has been named as the cause of permeability in the intestine, i.e. leaky gut.

## Irritable Bowel Syndrome --In depth

Irritable bowel syndrome (IBS) is a common disorder that affects your large intestine (colon). Irritable bowel syndrome commonly causes the following symptoms:

Symptoms

- Cramping
- Abdominal pain
- Bloating
- Pain
- Gas
- Diarrhea and /or constipation
- Despite these uncomfortable signs and symptoms, IBS doesn't cause permanent damage to your colon
- Flatulence

Irritable bowel syndrome (IBS) is a common disorder that affects your large intestine (colon).

Irritable bowel syndrome commonly causes cramping, abdominal pain, bloating gas, diarrhea, and constipation.

Despite these uncomfortable signs and symptoms, IBS doesn't cause permanent damage to your colon.

Most people with IBS find that symptoms improve as they learn to control their condition. Only a small number of people with irritable bowel syndrome have disabling signs and symptoms.

Fortunately, unlike more-serious intestinal diseases such as Ulcerative Colitis and Crohn's disease, Irritable Bowel Syndrome doesn't produce the same images on your x-rays or scans.

It doesn't demonstrate inflammation or changes in bowel tissue or increase your risk of colorectal cancer.

It has also been defined as a functional GI disorder where there is abdominal pain primarily, with some alteration of bowel habit.

Some people can have what is called diarrhea predominant, where you have abdominal pain. Often you might get the pain after a meal or when under stress.

## REPEATED VOMITING

If you have hereditary fructose intolerance, vomiting can trigger right after eating high-fructose foods. You can avoid undergoing this symptom by following a strict non-fructose diet. Avoid high-fructose corn syrup, table sugar or sucrose, confectionery or powdered sugar and honey. When drinking, avoid sodas, flavored water, sports drinks and sweetened milk, MayoClinic.com advises. Vegetables and fruits such as oranges, apples, and pears are known to have high natural fructose levels. Observing what you eat will promote longevity and good health.

## ABDOMINAL PAINS

Fructose intolerance can cause severe abdominal pain. The abdominal pain occurs soon after eating a meal that contained even a small amount of fructose. The best way to prevent the pain is managing your diet properly. A full understanding of the foods you can and cannot have is essential in managing fructose intolerance. If needed consult a registered dietitian for a proper diet regimen that suits your preference and lifestyle.

## HYPOGLYCEMIA

Hypoglycemia, or low blood sugar, is another symptom associated with hereditary fructose intolerance. Patients with fructose intolerance are unable to convert fructose into glucose, which is the main form of sugar in the bloodstream. As glucose levels drop, patients will develop hypoglycemia, which can manifest as fatigue, irritability, nausea, and loss of consciousness.

## WEIGHT GAIN

Fructose intolerance may interfere with your body's ability to metabolize glucose. The excess levels of glucose are then converted into fatty deposits and stored in adipose, or fat, tissue.

Therefore, fructose intolerance, by inhibiting glucose metabolism, can lead to weight gain, as noted in a May 2009 article in the "World Journal of Gastroenterology."

To avoid unwanted weight gain, you may need to adjust your diet and increase your exercise regimen. Consult your physician prior to starting a new workout routine.

Symptoms of HFI are as follows:

- Bloating (from fermentation in the small and large intestine)
- Diarrhea and/or constipation
- Flatulence
- Stomach Pain (as a result of muscle spasms...the intensity of which can vary from mild and chronic to acute but erratic)
- Nausea
- Vomiting (if great quantities are consumed)
- Early signs of clinical mental depression
- Fuzzy head
- Aching eyes
- Fatigue
- Rapid weight gain or loss
- Symptoms of hypoglycemia: sugar craving, tremor, fainting, and in severe cases convulsions or coma.

So...what is hereditary fructose (HFI) intolerance?

HFI is severe fructose intolerance due to genetic defects (aldolase B) mainly affecting children at the time of introduction of sugars, but also manifesting in adults. HFI and Fructose Malabsorbers have the same symptoms.

Fructose creates the metabolic disturbances, such as hypoglycemia, and permanent liver and kidney damage can ensue. In infants, the disease may be lethal due to seizures and coma.

After ingesting fructose, individuals may experience nausea, bloating, abdominal pain, diarrhea, vomiting, and low blood sugar (hypoglycemia).

Affected infants may fail to grow and gain weight at the expected rate (failure to thrive).

## Sensitivity

There is even sensitivity to the fructose component of sucrose, household sugar, as well as to infusions containing fructose. All forms of sucrose and fructose, and probably sorbitol, should be strictly avoided.

A positive family history of sugar intolerance or an aversion against sweets / candies is a useful clue. Diagnosis is by careful history taking, blood sampling for metabolic, liver and kidney disease, and, specifically, genetic testing. At present, not all forms of HFI can be identified using genetic blood tests.

First Hereditary Fructose Intolerance is rare and can be a life threatening condition.

This problem relates to a subnormal activity of Adolase B in the liver, kidney, and small bowel.

Symptoms only become present after the ingestion of Fructose.

Hereditary Fructose Intolerance (HFI) is generally diagnosed in young children but there are many substantiated cases of people reaching age 50 or older before it is diagnosed. I was adopted...so much of my family history was not known.

Since it is difficult to diagnosis in older people doctors don't generally perform, the necessary tests that are needed to correctly diagnosis these patients.

Anyone with who demonstrates the symptoms I have listed need to request that their doctor perform a Hydrogen Breath to rule out a Malabsorption problem.

Hereditary fructose intolerance is a genetic condition that affects a person's ability to digest the sugar fructose. Fructose is a simple sugar found primarily in fruits and vegetables. This is not an Allergy to fruits and vegetables it is much more. Processed foods contain huge levels of fructose, which creates a toxic mess for our digestive tract.

Repeated ingestion of fructose-containing foods can lead to liver and kidney damage. The liver damage can result in a yellowing of the skin and whites of the eyes (jaundice), an enlarged liver (hepatomegaly), and chronic liver disease (cirrhosis).

Continued exposure to fructose may result in seizures, coma, and ultimately death from liver and kidney failure due to the severity of symptoms experienced when fructose is ingested; most people with hereditary intolerance develop a dislike for fruits, juices, and other foods containing fructose.

Hereditary Fructose Intolerance should not be confused with a condition called Fructose Malabsorption.

In people with fructose malabsorption, the cells of the intestine cannot absorb fructose normally, leading to bloating, diarrhea or constipation, flatulence, and stomach pain.

Fructose malabsorption is thought to affect approximately 40 percent of individuals in the Western hemisphere; its cause is speculative, but the medical community acknowledges that Fructose issues are real.

How common is hereditary fructose intolerance?

The incidence of hereditary fructose intolerance is estimated to be 1 in 20,000 to 30,000 individuals each year worldwide.

What genes are related to hereditary fructose intolerance?

Mutations in the ALDOB gene cause hereditary fructose intolerance. The ALDOB gene provides instructions for making the aldolase B enzyme. This enzyme is found primarily in the liver and is involved in the breakdown (metabolism) of fructose so this sugar can be used as energy.

Aldolase B is responsible for the second step in the metabolism of fructose, which breaks down the molecule fructose-1-phosphate into other molecules called glyceraldehyde and dihydroxyacetone phosphate.

ALDOB gene mutations reduce the function of the enzyme, impairing its ability to metabolize fructose.

A lack of functional aldolase B results in an accumulation of fructose-1-phosphate in liver cells.

This buildup is toxic, resulting in the death of liver cells over time. In addition, the molecules produced from the breakdown of fructose-1-phosphate are needed in the body.

The breakdown of dihydroxyacetone phosphate releases a phosphate group (a cluster of oxygen and phosphorus atoms) from this molecule.

Phosphate groups are used for a number of cell processes, including the production of adenosine triphosphate (ATP), the cell's main energy source, and the release of stored sugar in the liver.

Lack of functional aldolase B enzyme reduces the amount of dihydroxyacetone phosphate, leading to fewer phosphate groups available for use in the body.

The death of liver cells and reduced number of phosphate groups lead to hypoglycemia, liver dysfunction, and other features of hereditary fructose intolerance.

Testing

Let me explain the hydrogen breath test (HBT) it is used to diagnose the presence of intolerance to dietary sugars, such as lactose, fructose, or sorbitol. The testing begins by having the patient drink a solution made up of the suspected substance.

If the intolerance exists the individual does not digest the sugar in the small intestine, the substance will make its way to the large intestine and be fermented by bacteria in the colon.

The by-product of this fermentation is hydrogen, which is then measured with a breath test administered several hours after the ingestion of the suspected substance.

If no such intolerance exists, the substance is thought to be digested in the small intestine, and there is no rise in breath hydrogen upon testing.

The hydrogen breath test may also be performed to assess the presence of SIBO (small intestine bacteria overgrowth *** see note ***). For SIBO testing, the breath test is administered sooner than when ruling out sugar intolerance, following the theory that the substance is being acted upon by bacteria found within the small intestine.

You are asked to drink, within a set time, a liquid solution containing a measured amount of powdered fructose.

You are then free to walk about but must report to the lab at specified intervals over a three-hour period when you are asked to blow into, and fill with your breath, a small plastic bag. These collected breath samples are analyzed for the gases of hydrogen and methane.

Recall that bowel bacteria ferment the fructose. This fermented fructose escapes as gas from your body in the form of flatulence as well as in your exhaled air.

If high concentrations of hydrogen or methane are found in your breath samples, this then is indicative of poor fructose absorption by the small bowel.

Testing for Intolerance

There are six types of test to detect if you have a dietary Intolerance issue.

- Glucose Breath Test to rule out Bacterial Overgrowth
- Lactose Breath Test to test for intolerance to milk and milk products
- Fructose Breath Test to determine intolerance to fructose
- Sucrose Breath Test if indicated from physical and oral history
- 3C stable Radioisotope; Breath tests for children and pregnant women. And Also, Uric Acid Levels

The Augusta doctor and his colleagues have worked to standardize the fructose breath test.

They have found a test solution of 25 grams of fructose allows them to identify those people having poor fructose absorption.

It is hard to believe that such a simple test, which can make a huge difference for millions of people, is not readily available. Part of the problem is many GI doctors are not well informed about the need for breath testing. Further, many GI centre's do not have the equipment for conducting breath tests.

What to do? The Gastroparesis & Dysmotilities Association (GPDA's) recommendation: while it is valuable to be diagnosed for fructose malabsorption, it is more important to take responsibility for your own health and to act now!

There is absolutely no harm in cutting back on your overall fructose intake!

Actually, there is a tremendous amount to be gained in terms of better health overall, improved blood-lipid profile, better insulin sensitivity, weight loss, improved blood pressure, and so on.

How do people inherit hereditary fructose intolerance?

This condition is inherited in an autosomal recessive pattern, which means both copies of the gene in each cell have mutations.

The parents of an individual with an autosomal recessive condition each carry one copy of the mutated gene, but they typically do not show signs and symptoms of the condition.

I never experienced any problem until late in life...so if someone tells you that you would have had these problems earlier that is not true...as previously stated there are many documented cases of the diagnosis being made in individuals that were in there 50's or 60's.

Remember hereditary fructose intolerance is a genetic disorder: that can be diagnosed at any age and Fructose Malabsorption can affect thousands of individuals!

## TREATMENT

There is no known cure, but appropriate food choices will help. I have now informed you that only a small percentage of people suffer from HFI, but many people suffer from Fructose Malabsorption!

Personal note from the Author: I walked 4 miles a day only to gain or become more bloated and have my pain increase. You must know what you are dealing with and change your diet prior to exercising.

## REFERENCES

HFI Laboratory at Boston University: Specifics of HFI and Its Diagnosis

MayoClinic.com: High Fructose Foods; March 26, 2011

national Institute of Diabetes and Digestive and Kidney Diseases; Hypoglycemia; October 2008  Johns Hopkins University; Fructose Intolerance, Hereditary; Cassandra L. Kniffin April 2009  "World Journal of Gastroenterology"; Adult hereditary fructose intolerance; Mohamed Ismail Yasawy et al; May 2009  May 12, 2011 | By Joseph Pritchard  Article reviewed by Mia Paul Last updated on: May 12, 2011

Printed in Great Britain
by Amazon

27437540R00190